ATTENTION DEFICIT HYPERACTIVITY DISORDER (ADHD) WORKBOOK

BY

JAMES ABRAM

DISCLAIMER

All Erudition contained in this book is given for informational and educational purposes only. The author is not in any way accountable for any results or outcomes that emanate from using this material. Constructive attempts have been made to provide information that is both accurate and effective, but the author is not bound for accuracy or use/misuse of information.

FOREWORD

First, I will like to thank you for taking the first step of trusting me and deciding to purchase/read this life transforming eBook. Thanks for spending your time and resources on this material. I can assure you of exact blueprint I lay bare in the information manual you are currently reading. It has transformed lives, and I strongly believe it will equally transform your life too. All the information I presented in this Do-It-Yourself is easy to digest and practice.

TABLE OF CONTENTS

INTRODUCTION

ADHD, or attention deficit hyperactivity disorder, is a condition as a rule found in kids and young people, and once in a while in grown-ups. It is regularly connected with learning challenges, prompting an inability to arrive at the scholastic execution level anticipated. At any rate one kid in every study hall is preoccupied, hyperactive, or both, and around 3–5 percent of the young populace is. The reason is perplexing and some of the time dubious; summoning hereditary and natural elements. A relative, a parent or youngster, has an expected 80 percent history of ADHD, and a portion of the potential causes are gentle imperfections in mind development, untimely birth and anoxic injury, disease, and lethal nicotine and lead presentation. Reports of MRI confirmation of fundamental mind irregularities, electroencephalographic dysrhythmias, and away from of untimely cerebrum development after neurological assessment bolster a physiological reason for ADHD.

Families may see hyperactive conduct not long after birth or when the youngster begins strolling, yet the analysis is frequently delayed until an educator sees the homeroom's inability to focus, occupy and eager conduct. When in doubt, an underlying appraisal by the pediatric or family doctor is trailed by conferences with the pediatric nervous system specialist or therapist, a mental assessment and, where demonstrated, lab assessments.

Treatment requires clinical lodging, drugs, conduct change, and social treatment. In 80 percent of kids with ADHD, focal apprehensive energizers have a surprising valuable impact, helping them to think, diminish unsettling and restless conduct, and advance learning and memory. Utilized as an instructive guide in traditionalist portions and firmly managed by a doctor, energizer pharmaceutical items are liberated from serious symptoms. Elective medications can be useful, including diet, and visual and sound-related arrangement however seldom give the quick and perceptible aftereffects of pharmacotherapy.

Probably the hardest issue confronting patients with various incapacities requests and ailments is looking for the most ideal help. Everybody is aware of companions or family members who have gotten care from an in any case decent doctor, just later to discover from another specialist that the underlying analysis was erroneous or that the recommended methodology were inadequate or even unsafe. A few patients, or individuals from the family, fathom this inquiry by perusing what they can about their manifestations, searching for subtleties on the web or effectively "making a few inquiries" to gain from companions and colleagues. Governments and lawmakers in the zone of medicinal services are likewise cognizant that patients in need won't really get similar results — what they allude to as variety in human services practice.

Presently overall human services administrations are attempting to address this variety by actualizing proof based practice. This essentially implies with a particular issue, it is to everybody's greatest advantage that patients have the most forward-thinking and fruitful treatment. Medicinal services authorities have now recognized that it is critical to offer however much information as could reasonably be expected to human services clients, with the goal that they can put forth better decisions in a coordinated attempt to improve physical wellbeing and emotional wellness. This show, Treatments That Work, intends to accomplish only that. The easy to understand jargon distinguishes just the new and best medications for specific issues. To be remembered for this arrangement, every treatment plan, as dictated by a clinical warning board, must fulfill the best expectations of proof accessible. Thusly, when people experiencing these conditions or individuals from their families look for a master clinician who knows about these medicines and concurs that they are worthy, patients will have confidence that they will get the most ideal treatment. Obviously, just the human services supplier will decide for you on the right blend of medications.

CHAPTER ONE

Definition and Hisitory of ADHD

ADHD, the Attention-Deficit / Hyperactivity Disorder abbreviation, is the term used to characterize the actions of infants, teenagers, and some adults who are inattentive, easily distracted, abnormally overactive, and impulsive. ADHD is a neurobiological "syndrome" with a common known cause and not a "disease." A number of different causes were proposed as being the cause of ADHD. The treatment involves many different approaches including fields of medicine, neuro-psychology, education, and parenting. The disease is "heterogeneous."

Over more than a century, ADHD was known under different titles. This is not a modern phenomenon or a result of the dynamic and fast-moving world of this twentieth century. Heinrich Hoffman (1809–1874), a German doctor and poet, wrote about Fidgety, Philip, 1955, in the nineteenth century, who could not sit still. The poem depicts a child's normal actions with ADHD, living in days when children were less permissive to supervision than they currently are. A more strict behavioral regulation did not appear to prevent the hyperkinetic condition from developing.

Brain Damage Syndromes

In papers written in the British journal, Lancet (1902, 1904) and the Journal of the American Medical Association (1921), scientific reference to a related childhood behavioral condition dates back to the early twentieth century. Among the earliest studies, clinical abnormalities were associated with head injury and emerged as a result of encephalitis following the 1918 World War I influenza epidemic.

In later articles (Hohman, 1922; Ebaugh, 1923; Strecker and Ebaugh, 1924) the similarities of hyperkinetic activity following head trauma and that reported in children recovering from encephalitis were defined. Those authors found both distractible and overactive children. "Natural drivenness" was a term used to characterize behavioral dysfunction following epidemic encephalitis, and the underlying cause of brainstem damage was suggested (Kahn and Cohen, 1934). Following this definition of behavioral symptoms triggered by brain disease or injury, a number of accounts of behavioral syndromes with specific features associated with brain damage or dysfunction.

Alternative Terms for ADHD

To identify the hyperactive child with attention deficits and sometimes related learning disabilities, a number of different words were used. Some have described the signs (hyperactivity, inattentiveness), some point to the suspected cause (brain damage or dysfunction), and some, the behavior-related behavioral difficulties (perception and learning disorders). The list of names for this condition is long, nearly 40 in number and some examples are as follows:

- Hyperactive (hyperkinetic) child syndrome.

- Baby suffering from brain injury.

- Minimum damaged brain.

- Baby with a visual disorder.

- Attention deficits, motor / perception (DAMP).

None of these definitions are entirely adequate, since the signs and causes of the condition are various and complex. Hyperactivity is the most common and shocking symptom, but some kids have regular or even lower rates of activity (hypokinesis), the condition often conveyed by inattention and distractiveness. Subtle brain disorders, defects in vision, and learning disabilities are frequently associated with, but not invariable findings. The common term ADHD highlights the symptoms but minimizes the significance of potential underlying causes and associated complications in neurology and learning.

Evolution of Present Concept of ADHD

From the initial description and concept of a brain damage syndrome, starting with postencephalitic behavioral disorder, proceeding in 1922 to the brain-injured child (1947) and the perceptually disabled child (1963) and ending with minimal brain dysfunction, in 1966, the emphasis turned to symptoms when the American Psychiatric Association included the syndrome in its Diagnostic and Statitic Association.

The first feedback of the syndrome in DSM-II (1968) used the term childhood or adolescent hyperkinetic reaction. In 1980, two subtypes of an attention deficit disorder (ADD) syndrome were recognized by the DSM-III – ADD with hyperactivity and ADD without hyperactivity. In 1987, the DSM-III (DSM-III-R) was revised, using the term attention-deficit hyperactivity disorder (ADHD). Ultimately, in 1994, the DSM-IV also defines three diagnosis subtypes: the form ADHD-inattentive, the form ADHD-hyperactive-impulsive and the type ADHD-combined. For through subtype diagnosis a minimum number of requirements are needed.

Diagnostic Criteria for ADHD Subtypes

(1) ADHD Subtype inattentive, without hyperactivity. For at least six months, at least six of the following nine symptoms have been reported, and are frequently present during school or play activities:

1. Makes errors carelessly;
2. Can not keep an eye out;
3. Does not listen when addressed;
4. Fails to complete assignments;
5. Seems to be disorganised;
6. Avoids duties;
7. Loses objects;
8. Easily distraught;
9. Forgotten.

(2) Subtype Hyperactive-Impulsive ADHD.

For at least six months there have been six (or more) of the following symptoms: Hyperactivity:

1. Fidgety,
2. Leaves seat in classroom or table;
3. Overruns or overruns;
4. Cannot play calmly;
5. Just "on the go";

6. A lot of conversations. Impulse:

7. Blurts out answers to questions;

8. Unable to wait in line, or turn;

9. Interrupts sometimes.

(3) ADHD Combined type.

Criteria were present for at least 6 months for both the Inattentive and the Hyperactive-Impulsive forms.

The term In Partial Remission refers to older children and adolescents whose symptoms have diminished with age or medication, and no longer add up to the diagnostic number needed.

Further Diagnostic Criteria

- Typical medical signs of ADHD include a recurring pattern of irregular severity and frequency inattention and/or hyperactivity and impulsiveness.

- Signs would have emerged before age 7.

- Symptoms should be found in at least two settings (school, home, workplace, or office of physician or psychologist).

- Symptoms tend to affect learning, social or job functions.

- The symptoms of a mental condition such as depression, anxiety or personality disorder can not be explained.

Questionnaires completed by parents, schoolteachers, psychologists and physicians are used to arrive at the diagnosis. A neurological examination that uncovers signs of a subtle form of brain impairment or injury, and psychological assessments that indicate deficiencies in vision and learning abilities, can be additional supporting evidence, although these results are not necessary for ADHD diagnosis. There is no clear chemical or laboratory examination, although elevated blood lead levels, thyroid hormone deficiency, or other chromosomal abnormalities (fragile X disease) may rarely provide an explanation for the symptoms.

ADHD, a Continuum or Medical Syndrome

In one major twin study reported from Prince of Wales Hospital, Randwick, NSW and involving approximately 2000 families recruited from the Australian MRC Twin Registry, ADHD is treated as a continuum rather than a distinct medical condition. ADHD is defined as an inherited condition with a population-wide obligation and language, a deviance from an acceptable standard and not limited to an arbitrary number of symptoms or diagnostic criteria for DSM. The need for care and drugs depends on several factors and is subjective.

ADHD, a Medical Deficit or Social Deviance

Many skeptics claim that ADHD symptoms can be explained by a "standard" behavior change, a so-called boisterous infant, or a representation of our culture. Sociologists blame physicians for "medicalizing" signs that should be considered deviant behavior and adaptation to the social environment (Conrad, 1973, Conrad and Schneider, 1980);

The medical definition of deviant behavior has therapeutic benefits for the person, allowing less judgment among peers and adults and less social stigma. The baby with an ADHD diagnosis is no longer the classroom's "bad guy." He has a "illness," which includes daily medical visits to the nurse at lunchtime. The noisy and distracting conduct is not his responsibility. ADHD diagnosis is also used as an excuse for performing disorders and drug use, often putting pressure to bear on the justice system and demanding undeserved leniency.

According to the sociologists, the "medicalization" of ADHD accompanied the availability of a drug, methylphenidate, to regulate the deviant behaviour. Researchers conclude that if the paradoxical, quieting effect of stimulant drugs had not been identified the condition would not be known as an disease (Bradley, 1937). By identifying ADHD as a medical problem, we might be taking focus away from family, education, or other factors of probable underlying significance in the social setting.

Such claims are a significant reminder to physicians, parents, and teachers that the child's treatment of ADHD does not depend exclusively on the prescription of stimulant or other drugs. Treatment is "multimodal," including parental therapy, adjustment of child behavior, the acceptable size of the classroom the instructional methods, and medical care.

Prevalence of ADHD and Gender Factor

Around 5 percent of children and teens are affected, or at least one in each classroom. Boys are most commonly affected three to six times more than children. Some authorities estimated the prevalence at school children between 5 and 12 years of age to be as high as 10 percent, and even 20 percent. Another study estimated that the United States had a total of 3 million children with ADHD.

ADHD is recognized worldwide, but the prevalence reported varies in different countries, with less than 1 in 1000 in a 10- and 11-year-old study in the island of Wight, UK (Rutter et al., 1970). The accuracy and comparison of these figures is influenced by the research population age, patient selection variation and lack of consensus on the concept of diagnostic criteria.

In a study of 8,000 children in a Tennessee county at Vanderbilt University, Nashville, TN, of ratings completed by 400 teachers, ADHD prevalence rates were higher when using the latest diagnostic criteria specified in DSM-IV compared to DSM-III-R criteria. Prevalence rates for ADHD using DSM-III-R were 7% and DSM-IV were 11%, an improvement of 57%. The in-attentional (AD) subtype of ADHD was 5%, the hyperactive-impulsive (H-I) group 2.5% and the overall group 3.5%. Boys outnumbered girls with the ADHD-HI ratio 4:1 and the ADHD-AD ratio 2:1.

Age of Onset of ADHD

Some signs should be present by the age of seven years according to the DSM-IV guidelines for the diagnosis of ADHD. Hyperactivity is recognized more commonly when the child begins school at around four or five years of age, although many parents complain of extreme motor restlessness in infancy. In fact, due to excessive fetal movements during pregnancy, some mothers had expected the birth of a hyperactive child.

The environment is also affected by the time symptoms begin. Upon entering a structured environment, such as a school classroom, a child who is slightly anxious at home or in the doctor's office can become hyperactive and distractable. As in private tutoring, the child will work relatively well on a one-to - one, student-teacher ratio, whereas the signs of ADHD may quickly become evident in a large class of students. Parents are often dismayed at school records, as symptoms can be less noticeable in the home setting.

ADHD from an Educational Perspective

Many research (e.g., Barkley et al., 1990) have observed children with ADHD attaining lower grades in academic subjects than their peers. More recently this pattern has been observed among children with ADHD symptoms reported by teachers (Merrell & Tymms, 2001; McGee et al., 2002; Merrell & Tymms, 2005a). These children, detected at school at the end of their first year, have at this stage substantially lower reading and mathematics performance than children with no reported behavioral issues.

They fell even further behind by the end of primary school, especially those children with inattentional symptoms. Wolraich and colleagues also say that carelessness is a central component in low academic performance (Wolraich et al., 2003). Use rating scales based on the diagnostic criteria described in DSM-IV-TR, the proportion of children identified in the classroom by their teachers as inattentional, hyperactive and/or impulsive was reported to be between 8.1 and 17 percent. A later study by Wolraich and colleagues (2004) showed that a higher estimate of 25 percent of their pupils with a high risk of ADHD was provided by teachers screening of elementary pupils.

Once children begin school, aged 4 or 5, their teachers will be very well positioned to recognise the symptoms of ADHD. The school setting problems are likely to make such difficulties more evident, and teachers who are trained in observing a wide variety of children's behaviour, can pick up on them. Nevertheless, Bailey (2006) warns that inattentional, hyperactive and impulsive behavior may be a reaction to the school environment's demands and constraints, and it is necessary to note that this could be the case for some children. Theoretically, once children with signs of ADHD have been reported, further assessment should be performed and interventions can be placed in place at an early stage, while studies by Tymms and Merrell did not support screening. Early intervention can be effective in minimizing behavioral problems and adverse effects, and the better the sooner it is introduced. O'Shaughnessy and colleagues (2003) also proposed that organized school-wide detection and behavioral adjustment strategies for children improve the probability of enhancing their outcomes. Although many studies have found that classroom-based approaches have a positive impact on the actions of children with ADHD and, to a lesser extent, on their academic progress (Purdie et al., 2002), teachers in

England are currently not routinely qualified to use these teaching and management strategies in classrooms.

All children and youth, including those with ADHD, are entitled to a school experience that includes a comprehensive, balanced and appropriate curriculum, including the National Curriculum, adequately differentiated by their needs. This has consequences for initial teacher preparation and professional growth within the company. Additionally, a whole school approach to encouraging good conduct outside and within the classroom is important, and training will apply to non-teaching staff members. Several studies have shown that the perceived competence of teachers and student teachers in the management of children with ADHD in the classroom is variable and associated with their expertise and experience in the profession. There is still a lack of training, as demonstrated by the report of the Education and Skills Select Committee on Special Educational Needs (House of Commons Education and Skills Committee, 2006), which recommended that' the government should dramatically increase its expenditure in the preparation of its employees so that all workers, including teachers, are fully equipped and prepared for training.

Economic Cost of ADHD

The actual reported prevalence of children and young people with ADHD in the United Kingdom is 3.62% in boys and 0.85% in girls (Ford et al., 2003). Based on these estimates and national population statistics (Office for National Statistics, 2007), it can be estimated that in England and Wales about 210,000 children aged 5 to 18 years are affected by ADHD, but only a minority of them may seek or obtain medical care (Sayal et al., 2002, 2006a). Across England and Wales, children with ADHD have been reported to inflict substantial burdens on health, social and educational services, hitting £ 23 million for initial specialist assessment, and £ 14 million annually for follow-up treatment, excluding medication. Those estimates do not reflect health and social care expenses borne by people with ADHD.

The total annual cost of prescription stimulants and other medications for ADHD in England in 2006 was nearly £ 29 million, a rise of 20 percent from the previous year (NHS Health and Social Care Information Centre, 2006; NHS Information Centre, 2007). The cost increase is partly due to the increased number of people being treated, and partly to a change in prescribing toward more complex formulations of MR. Schlander (2007) projected that ADHD pharmacotherapy expenditure on children and youth in England will reach £ 78 million in 2012, owing to an increase in the number of diagnosed cases, increased pharmacotherapy acceptance and strength, and higher unit costs of new drugs.

Nonetheless, the estimated £ 29 million annual cost of prescription ADHD drugs in England is rather low compared to the annual cost of prescribed drugs for other chronic conditions such as depression (£ 292 million) and diabetes (£ 562 million) (The Information Centre, 2006).

UK statistics on ADHD's economic costs are limited; since US figures refer to a very different service delivery pattern, they can not be generalized with the UK. Costs in the US have risen over the years due to an ever-increasing clinician recognition rate, with paediatricians identifying from 1.4 percent of children in 1979 to 9.2 percent in 1996. Birnbaum and colleagues (2005) reported that, in 2000 rates, the overall expense of ADHD in the US was $31.6 billion, using a prevalence of 8% for youth, 4% for girls, 5% for male adults and 3.5% for female adults. For this expense, only 5 percent ($1.6 billion) were specifically related to the diagnosis of the condition; the remainder were other healthcare costs for children and adults with ADHD ($12.1 billion or 38 percent), healthcare costs for family members with ADHD ($14.2 billion or 45 percent), and economic losses for adults with ADHD and adult family members with ADHD ($3.7 percent).

Such figures reflect excess costs, i.e. extra expenses for people with ADHD and their families, over and above the respective expenses of equivalent individual controls.

Pelham and his colleagues (2007) reported an estimated annual cost of ADHD for children and youth at around $14,600 per individual in 2005 prices (ranging from $12,000 to $17,500), consisting of healthcare costs (18 percent), education costs (34 percent), as well as crime- and delinquency costs (48 percent). Using a prevalence rate of 5 per cent, the authors calculated a total expense of $42.5 billion (range from $36 to $52.5 billion) for children and people with ADHD in the US.

In the United States, children with ADHD have been found to face comparable healthcare costs to children with asthma and considerably higher than those of children without ADHD. This cost differential was found to be linked to a higher number of encounters with general practitioners (GPs) and ambulatory mental health facilities, emergency room visits, and hospitalizations. In addition, children with ADHD are more likely to experience other coexisting medical disorders such as behavioral disorder, oppositional defiant disorder, and depression, and so on, relative to children without ADHD, which greatly increases the use of health care facilities and related costs. Children with ADHD are also much more likely to have learning difficulties and to face higher educational costs than children without ADHD; these costs may include the costs of special education and the costs of providing medication to children with ADHD either to a school nurse or to office personnel. Adults with ADHD also face high healthcare costs compared to matched adults without ADHD, given the comparatively low ADHD diagnosis levels in this age group, estimated at about 25 per cent in the US.

Adults with ADHD are more likely to have a comorbid diagnosis of asthma, depression, anxiety, bipolar disorder, antisocial personality disorder, and alcohol or drug abuse which further leads to medical expenses. However, even after accounting for the effects of coexisting conditions, it was found that adults with ADHD had higher inpatient and outpatient costs, as well as the cost of prescription drugs. A person with ADHD in the US had an average annual expense of $5,600 in premiums in 2001, versus $2,700 for a matched person with no ADHD. However, it should be remembered that adult ADHD entails lower health-care costs per person relative to other medical conditions, such as depression or diabetes. The prevalence of ADHD in adults is associated with increased economic losses due to absenteeism and declines in job efficiency, in addition to the rise in healthcare costs.

The carers and families of people with ADHD often bear considerable costs in terms of out - of-pocket expenses as well as productivity losses due to decreased ability to work and absenteeism, in addition to affected individuals. Additionally, families with children with ADHD have a major emotional burden, which includes strained family relationships (parent-child or sibling interactions), anxiety and worry parenting, and marital conflict. Additional costs are correlated with higher injury rates.

From the above study, it is clear that ADHD is associated with significant financial and emotional costs to the healthcare system, educational services, carers and friends, and to the entire community. Providing effective treatment would improve the quality of life of people with ADHD, their carers and their families, while at the same time reducing the financial and psychological effects of ADHD on society.

CHAPTER TWO

Brief Overview of the Executive Functions

In this culture, life as an adult is difficult so those with poor executive functions can fail and stand out. They will have trouble managing all of life's information and making "rational" choices (i.e. choices that more favor the future than the present). Many adults with untreated ADHD are considered reckless or inexperienced, since at the moment they appear to respond too quickly and lose sight of the greater picture. This is something that society expects and forgives of children, but not of adults. Because of these challenges in handling the thousand and one aspects of daily life, people with ADHD spend a great deal of time trying to keep it all together and avoid catastrophe. Putting out fires needs a lot more energy than stopping them. This reactive lifestyle is much more intense than one that other adults without ADHD have been living.

They expect adults to be able to show self-control and do not require as much help from others. Because individuals with ADHD tend to make themselves do the right thing at the right moment, parents and romantic partners frequently step in and have such cognitive functions and prevent their loved one from heading too far off the rails — for example, by reminding her of coming meetings, arranging her stuff or avoiding impulsive purchases. Alternatively, she could consider devices that can do the job for her — for instance, setting up automatic debits to avoid having to remember sending out the bills or using a mobile to remind her of coming meetings.

A Brief Overview of the Executive Functions

Various scholars have drawn up many different lists of executive functions. I find that the reaction inhibition theory of Russell Barkley is the most detailed and practical of these, and the theory of executive functions I explore in this workbook is an outcome of his work. His theory is extremely comprehensive and interesting, but it requires much more knowledge to handle your everyday life than you need to know. And I've taken out the pieces that are most relevant to your everyday life — the parts that not only illustrate why certain issues are so hard for you but also set the stage for the successful approaches that we're going to explore.

The Executive Functions Develop Over Time

The creation of the executive functions is part of the natural brain maturation cycle. As the neurons grow and attach through our brains we learn all kinds of skills, from walking to talking to thinking about abstract concepts. Generally speaking, the skills of adults are more advanced than those of children as our brains begin to mature in our 30s.

As with most growth, a combination of genetics and environmental exposure guids this process. Our genes provide us with a range of possibilities, and then experience shapes the genetic expression.

A lot of conditions happen in the case of ADHD. It's one of the most inheritable disorders in all mental health. Much like there are other talents flowing in families (such as being a successful athlete or having an ear for music), so there are genes that influence the executive functions and ADHD neurons involved.

Yeah, your ADHD isn't the product of your parents not doing enough good work — and there's not anything your parents might have done differently to alleviate your ADHD symptoms. You can only blame your parents for your upbringing when it comes to your ADHD, but if you have children of your own you may want to avoid that line of reasoning.

Summaries of the Executive Functions

In this workbook, I have included brief summaries of each of the executive functions we will discuss. Ideally this will make these often amorphous ideas feel more real and linked more easily to your everyday life. In the exercises we will become very realistic, but it helps to begin with a good understanding of the theory.

Working Memory: The Brain's RAM

We are actively using working memory to keep in mind details while we recall what has just happened, link it to long-term memories and look forward into the future. Working memory and attention function very closely together, because working memory retains what we attend to. People with ADHD tend to have blinky working memories which lead to a variety of daily problems.

Sense of Time: It Can't Be 5:00 Already

People with ADHD have trouble tracking the passing of time and preparing accordingly, a skill which is very necessary in the busy world of today. As a result, they appear to spend too much time on other tasks and don't schedule enough time on others. This leads to their well-known time-management issues and to getting places on time.

Remembering to Remember: It's All About Timing

We all have hundreds of little (and not so little) things in our busy lives to recall doing over the course of a day, such as phone calls and appointments or returning to something after an interruption. People with ADHD have considerable difficulty in recalling these things at the right time, often fully forgetting or just remembering when it's too late.

Emotional Self-Control: Having Feelings

Individuals with ADHD without acting on them appear to feel and express their emotions more intensely than others do, and are more affected by their emotions than most individuals are. This then inhibits their ability to see in the moment beyond their feelings and take into account the experiences of others.

Self-Activation: Starting Then Finishing

Everyone needs to use some willpower to get on with tedious activities but those with ADHD have a much steeper hill to climb. As a result, they appear to procrastinate before they are pushed into action by the burden of an imminent deadline.

Hindsight and Forethought: Using the Past and Future to Guide the Present

This time we are using the insights from previous encounters to make better decisions. We are also thinking strategically about the possible results of various acts to select the strategy with the highest chances of success. People with ADHD tend to respond too fast at the moment, and don't make the time to consider the past or think about the future, so they're more likely to make less desirable choices.

While we can consciously choose to handle circumstances in certain ways, many of the executive functions, including breathing, work without conscious knowledge. If you watch little kids talk themselves through a challenging task, they're kind of verbalizing their executive functions — for example, gently explaining to themselves what they're supposed to be doing or guiding themselves along the way. Eventually it is natural and we don't have to worry about it as much, but we may also find that we still become very deliberate in difficult circumstances while using our executive functions.

Although I am talking about different executive functions, keep in mind that they are constantly communicating with each other and that the distinctions between them can be quite blurred. Don't hold on exactly what executive function is at work in any given situation. The purpose of this workbook is to make it clear and practical in your daily life, which often requires a bit of simplification.

Response Inhibition: It Starts with Stopping

The funny thing about executive functions is that they are very well used by people with ADHD — except when they don't. In fact, this inconsistency is a characteristic of ADHD (if someone is suffering consistently, then the guilty party is possibly something other than ADHD). So how can we describe that people with ADHD often do very well but make very basic mistakes at other times?

This is where the principle of Barkley's inhibition response comes into play. Unlike simpler life-forms that automatically respond to environmental stimuli, humans may hold back an automatic response to the world around them (as well as their inner world of thoughts and feelings). This critical stopping capacity provides a pause that allows them to think about the various answer choices and then select the right one. This typically occurs within a split second. An example is almost subconsciously deciding to ignore someone's sound dropping a pen when you're working on your screen (i.e. not getting distracted) or keeping your attention on what someone is saying before they end up talking (i.e. not interrupting impulsively).

The secret to good decision taking is the tiny little delay, as it gives time to do their thing to the executive functions. In the small space between stimulus and response the executive functions work. People with ADHD have trouble stopping long enough to establish the break, so they don't use their executive functions as consistently or as efficiently as others. As a consequence, they get overwhelmed, forget things, and jump without looking, etc .— the ADHD symptoms you so well know.

That explains why people with ADHD are not always doing what they think they should be doing. Since they have difficulty creating the pause which allows them time to make a well-considered decision, they are more vulnerable to being affected by something happening around them. They have difficulty filtering out external and internal information, so they respond to what is "wrong." An example is to answer the phone and engage in a long conversation instead of getting ready to leave the house on time. It may sound like poor judgement, but what really happens is that these other factors have too great an effect on the decision-making of the ADHD person, and it makes a less than ideal option. It's not poor judgement, but they didn't hesitate long enough in these knee-jerk responses to objectively judge. This is why those dreaded questions of "why did/didn't you… lead to such unconvincing answers along the lines of "I don't know. I really didn't think about it, 'which is pretty true actually. Our thoughts had not slowed long enough to get an opportunity to think about it.

Since people with ADHD response inhibition problems appear to make them so vulnerable to being excessively affected by external and internal stimuli, many of the techniques to help them concentrate more effectively on increasing the intensity of the desired stimulus or reducing the intensity of less desirable stimulus so they do the right thing at that level. A beeping warning that tells the person to leave for a meeting, for example, overrides the emphasis on what else he was doing.

Medicines (as well as Cogmed Working Memory Training and likely neurofeedback) function directly by improving the brain's capacity to establish the pause, thus eliminating the pause-induced impact. That's also why admonitions to "just try harder" don't work — they neglect the underlying issue people with ADHD have difficulty generating the moment of pause to try harder in. It's like explaining to someone who wants glasses that she just has to remember to look harder. It is a power issue, not desire. The frustrating aspect is that people with ADHD typically have the ability to do the actual task (like paying the bills) but are not as good at the simple ability to establish the delay, so they don't get to the actual task.

Note this pause when we talk at length about executive functions and run through the exercises in Section II, as this is the tripping point for many executive-functioning malfunctions. And the approaches that perform best are those that take this into account.

Neurology and Psychology

I prefer to make a somewhat simplistic distinction between neurologically driven behaviors and psychologically driven ones. We cannot distinguish them entirely from each other but there are moments when it is helpful to think about these two different contributions. A lot of ADHD is psychological but lifetime of ADHD creates a lot of psychology.

I prefer to think of working memory, sense of time, and prospective memory as more simply cognitive when it comes to executive functions, with less of a psychological impact. Our psychological state can influence how we use these executive functions, but they work mostly without our conscious consciousness.

However, more psychology is interwoven into the neuronal working through emotional self-control, self-activation and intuition and forethought. For example, if you feel like you are constantly getting your family's short end of the stick, you are less likely to exhibit good emotional control when something comes up with them.

If you feel like you have some pretty good strategies in place but things just aren't rolling for you, figuring out some stuff might even be worth meeting with a therapist. I'm certainly not saying that ADHD's main traits will be fixed by counseling, but it can be helpful for the miss. Only make sure you find a person who is pretty knowledgeable about ADHD. I know, finding someone who knows the stuff can take some real looks, but if you do, it's worth it.

Fallout from Executive Function Weaknesses

The deficiencies in the executive function involved in ADHD contribute to the symptoms you know so well, such as irritation, forgetfulness or impulsiveness. The information-processing functions which underlie ADHD cause the symptoms, so we get to the root of the problem by talking about the executive functions.

CHAPTER THREE

The Causative Factors of ADHD

ADHD is a highly heritable disease but, in addition to genetic causes, often inherited and environmental influences that may be prone to prevention or alternative treatment are discovered. The causes of ADHD can be classified as idiopathic, naturally arising from an unknown cause, symptomatic and secondary to a structural abnormality of the brain, or from family and assumed genetics. Most ADHD cases are idiopathic, or cause uncertain. A delay in nervous system development or maturation is often suggested as an explanation for ADHD, particularly for children with moderate or "soft" neurological deficits.

Etiological Classification

Sometimes, the etiologies of ADHD are defined by the time they occur:

(1) Prenatal;
(2) Perinatal; and
(3) Postnatal.

The syndrome may be inherited and family, or acquired and environmentally friendly. Rarely, the root cause of ADHD is chromosomal disorder.

Prenatal factors include neurological developmental deficiency, maternal anemia, pregnancy toxemia, drug and cocaine misuse, and smoke from tobacco. Many environmental factors that are often suspected include exposure to arsenic, water and diet PCBs and pesticides, lack of iodine, and hypothyroidism. Birth season may be a risk factor, and exposure to viral infections, especially influenza and viral exanthema, has been associated with ADHD diagnosis in the first trimester of pregnancy or at the time of birth.

Perinatal etiological causes include: premature birth, breech delivery, anoxic-encephalopathy, hemorrhage of the cerebrum, meningitis, and encephalitis.

Postnatally the child may have had a head injury, meningitis, encephalitis, repeated otitis media attacks, or low blood sugar. Drugs used in the treatment of childhood disorders, asthma and epilepsy, often induce or intensify hyperactive behavior and result in delays in attention and learning. Diet's role in causing ADHD is uncertain, but ingestion of food additives and saccharosis, lack of omega-3 fatty acids, and allergies to certain foods are sometimes important. Potential causes and occasionally, thyroid hormone deficiency is associated with ADHD are known as lack of iron in the diet and anemia (Millichap, 2008). An abnormality of sensory feedback soothed by oral potassium is suggested in a 9-year-old boy with symptoms of sensory overstimulation and potassium sensitivity as a novel cause of ADHD.

Evidence for a Neurological Basis for ADHD

The neurological or anatomical theory of hyperactivity and ADHD is focused on various animal laboratory trials, neurological and electroencephalographic (EEG) experiments, and brain magnetic resonance imaging (MRIs). Studies of positron emission tomography (PET), revealing improvements in the glucose metabolism in the brain's frontal lobes, point to a localized cerebral abnormality in adults who have been hyperactive since childhood.

Neurological "soft" symptoms are characteristic of right-sided frontal cortical lesions, including motor impersistence (incapacity to maintain postures or movements), distractibility (incapacity to maintain attention), and careful control and reaction inhibition. The largest number and degree of hyperactive behavioral responses derive from frontal cerebral lesions and their associations with the basal ganglia or striate cortex. The right prefrontal cortex plays a part in regulating attention and inhibiting responses, while the basal ganglia are involved in motor regulation and behavioral responses. In children with ADHD, distractibility and impulsivity represent deficits in response inhibition.

Injury or irregular development in regions of the brain other than the frontal lobes can also be associated with ADHD syndrome and language and social competencies deficiency. For children with temporal lobe lesions, cognitive dysfunction and ADHD are identified, and in such cases a link with the front striatal circuitry is likely.

In 4 children with bilateral medial temporal lobe (hippocampus) sclerosis, associated with severe epilepsy starting in early childhood, deficits of cognitive function, language growth, and social skills were identified at Duke University Medical Center, Durham, NC. MRI displayed irregular signals and hippocampal volume loss of 25 per cent.

In some patients of childhood, temporal lobe arachnoid cyst is identified in combination with ADHD. The diagnosis of this relationship and condition, though rare, points to the possible significance of prenatal factors in the cause of ADHD. The cause of arachnoid cyst is typically undetermined, but trauma, bleeding, or virus infection is likely to cause damage to the fetal brain. In patients with elevated intracranial pressure and complicated headaches or seizures, care may include surgery to remove the cyst, but other, more restrictive interventions may usually control the symptoms.

Analyzes of brain volume by MRI. Measurements of different brain structures using quantitative MRI techniques have revealed changes in corpus callosum size, decreased volume of right prefrontal cortex and basal ganglia, smaller cerebellar vermis, and smaller cerebral volume. In children with ADHD, MRI measurements of the right prefrontal cortex and basal ganglia correlate with response inhibition and task success. Decreased cerebral volumes can explain lower scores on IQ tests in some children with ADHD.

At the Western Psychiatric Institute, University of Pittsburgh, PA, MRI volumetric study revealed differences between task performance and prefrontal and caudate volume in the right hemisphere in 26 children with ADHD as opposed to 26 normal controls. Only right prefrontal measures correlated with inhibition-including response efficiency.

In the ADHD group, quantitative MRI studies in 46 right-handed boys with ADHD and 47 matched healthy controls at the National Institute of Mental Health, Bethesda, MD, found a smaller cerebellar vermis, especially involving subsequent inferior lobules. Within ADHD a malfunction of the cerebello-thalamo-prefrontal circuit is postulated.

Localized cerebral hemisphere and cerebellar developmental abnormalities in ADHD are associated with impaired striatal-cerebellar frontal activity, and often with stimulant response.

At the University of California, Irvine, volumetric MRI brain analysis showed smaller volumes of localized hemispheric structures in 15 male ADHD infants, compared to 15 normal controls. Smaller left basal ganglia (specifically caudate nucleus) was associated with stimulant drug response while non-responders had reversed caudate asymmetry.

MRI tests of the head of the caudate nucleus at the University of Barcelona, Spain associated with neuropsychological disorders and behavioral problems in 11 adolescents with ADHD. The ADHD group had a larger right caudate nucleus, and the usual L > R caudate asymmetry had been reversed.

The multiple anatomical sites of brain damage or lesion that are often found in children with ADHD that account for the syndrome's varying symptoms and complications.

Based on cerebral blood flow, EEG tests and volumetric MRI measurements, a frontal-motor cortex disconnection syndrome, or "lazy" frontal lobe, is proposed in ADHD. This idea is derived from the frontal lobe's role as an excessive motor activity regulator, with children with ADHD having disinhibited motor activity. Methylphenidate's calming effect may be attributed to a relaxing effect on the frontal lobe inducing motor inhibition.

EEG ADHD and Anomalies. For children with ADHD with varying frequencies, epileptiform discharges in the EEG are recorded from 6% to 53%. The reason for an EEG in ADHD includes:

(1) A history of seizures;
(2) Repeated "daydreaming;"
(3) A history of brain trauma, encephalitis, or meningitis; and
(4) A reference to stimulant therapy in patients with an epileptic background or family history. A proportion of ADHD patients are more vulnerable to seizures, based on EEG evidence.

Computerized power spectral analysis for EEG statistical analysis reveals that boys aged 9–12 with ADHD have increased theta (4.75 Hz) and decreased beta 1 (12.75–21 Hz) activity relative to age- and grade-level controls (Mann, 1992). The increased theta is located in the frontal and central locations, and in posterior and temporal areas, the beta decreased.

EEG results from 184 boys with a combination form of ADHD showed three distinct EEG clusters or subtypes of children distinguished by

(a) Increased slow wave activity and rapid wave deficiencies;

(b) Increased theta of high amplitude with beta deficiencies; and

(c) An excess beta community.

As far as EEG profile, kids with ADHD don't comprise a homogenous class. Quantitative EEG information in kids with ADHD may give more precise proportions of mindful issues than are presently accessible from abstract polls or rating scales. Inconstancy of EEG attributes must be recollected whether soon the EEG is utilized as a dependable analytic technique for ADHD.

Impact of Genetic Factors in Etiology of ADHD

Families would also admit that during infancy, fathers and mothers were hyperactive or had a learning problem. They will also dispute any childhood behaviour or attention issues, despite being unable to sit quietly during the consultation. It's not unusual to have a history of relatives and cousins diagnosed with ADHD who have had a positive reaction to stimulant medication.

It is hard to prove the strong difference between the influence of nature and diet in the cause of ADHD, and both the genetic and acquired factors are significant. The cause may be solely genetic in some cases, in others, primarily acquired and environmental, and in others, a mixture of both. Epidemiologists use many methods to demonstrate the function of genetic factors as opposed to environmental influences.

(1) **ADHD predominance in various geographic, ethnic, or racial populaces.**

In an investigation of 145 kids determined to have ADHD at the Shaare Zedek Medical Center, Jerusalem, Israel, young men dwarfed young ladies by 3:1, 30 percent had kin with learning inabilities contrasted with only 7 percent among control kids without ADHD, and 34 percent were of North African root, an ethnic gathering present in only 12 percent of the number of inhabitants in Jerusalem. A familial-hereditary factor right now patients was reflected by the dominance of guys, the expanded pervasiveness of learning troubles in kin, and an ethnic-related inclination to ADHD.

(2) **Risk of ADHD in first-degree family members (guardians, kin, and offspring) of patients with ADHD contrasted with everyone:**

Of the 457 first degree family members of youngsters and teenagers alluded to the Child Psychiatry Program, Massachusetts General Hospital, Boston, the danger of ADD, just as introverted and temperament issue was generously higher than among regular controls.

(3) **Twin investigations:** One may liken indistinguishable, monozygous (MZ) twins with brotherly, dizygous (DZ) twins. IF hereditary elements are noteworthy, both MZ twins are influenced (concordant), while for common kin, concordance in DZ twins is lower, and indistinguishable. For ADHD inquire about, DZ twins must be of a similar sex, in light of the fact that there is a male prevalence. A case of the job of natural impacts in the advancement of ADHD is how much MZ twins might be conflicting (i.e., just one influenced).

An assessment of 10 sets of twins, at any rate one of which had the hyperactive condition, found that every one of the four sets of MZ twins were dependable, while just one of six sets of DZ were concordant. The twins at the MZ were all young men. A hereditary reason for ADHD is affirmed by this exploration.

The Minnesota Twin Family Report, including 576 twin young men matured 11 and 12, and educator and maternal examination survey, confirmed the job of hereditary factors in the treatment of ADHD subtypes of both obliviousness and hyperactivity-hastiness. Natural conditions had less etiological supporters of ADHD.

Twin studies using ADHD interview testing at the UCLA School of Medicine, Los Angeles, CA, revealed 79 percent concordance in 37 monozygotic twins, compared to 32 percent in 37 same-sex dizygotic twins. ADHD is a genetic disease with a prevalence five to six times higher in the first-degree genetic compared to the general population. ADHD proband relatives have increased levels of comorbid conditions, especially oppositional and behavioral disorders, anxiety, mood disorders and learning disabilities. Studies of adoption endorse both a genetic basis for ADHD as well as environmental causes.

(4) **Influence of environmental upbringing among MZ twins:**In foster homes, comparison of MZ twins reared together versus MZ twins reared apart helps epidemiologists to differentiate genetic impact from environmental influences within a population. It is also important to assess the occurrence of ADHD in the biologic or the adoptive relatives or half-sibs.

In a sample of full sibs and half-sibs of 14 children with limited brain impairment (ADHD), all born in foster homes, 50% of full sibs versus 14% of half-sibs had hyperactive behavior and care deficiencies (Safer, 1969). Such results were more in support of genetic than environmental causes in the development of ADHD although the research was skewed by a higher frequency of premature and neonatal problems among the complete sibs, environmental factors reported to development ADHD.

Chromosomal Anomalies Associated with ADHD

Chromosomal syndromes are uncommon in patients suffering from ADHD. They include unstable syndromes such as X, velocardiofacial deletion (22Q.11.2), Williams, Turner and Prader-Willi, and type 1 neurofibromatoses (Moore et al., 1996). One girl had a sex chromosome aneuploidy (47.XXX) and one boy had a permutation-sized allele for fragile X in a study of 100 children (64 boys) with ADHD (combined type) and normal intelligence, but none displayed the complete mutation. Tests were negative for microdeletion 22q11.2. Routine chromosome study in children with ADHD is not commonly recommended in the absence of clinical symptoms or a family history.

Molecular Genetic Studies

The studies above draw attention to the role of genetic factors in the cause of ADHD. Proving an inherited predisposition is also needed to recognize a particular metabolic or enzyme marker. Catecholaminergic candidate-focused studies affirm the presence of the dopamine receptor and dopamine transporter genes (DAT1). Deficits in frontal-striatal circuits moduled by dopamine are associated with ADHD subtypes. The relationship between dopamine deficits and fetal and perinatal stress can explain the mechanism of ADHD's environmental etiology (Swanson et al., 2007). Premature birth, which is complicated by susceptibility to cerebral ischemia, may lead to increased availability of dopamine receptors, impaired dopaminergic transmission and subsequent development of ADHD.

Twin experiments have shown evidence of environmental mediators in ADHD. Affected twins are more prone to risk factors like maternal smoking, lower birth weights and delayed growth and development compared to unaffected co-twins. Interaction between genes and the environment is increasingly recognized as an important role in the etiology and development of ADHD, with certain genes (e.g., DAT1) influencing individual sensitivity to etiological factors.

Environmental Factors in Etiology

While sometimes speculative, the evidence for environmental and acquired influences is far better than the genetic data in the quest for causes of ADHD. Maternal smoking and nicotine, exanthema, maternal iron deficiency, breech conveyance, rashness, low birth weight, hypoxic-ischemic-encephalopathy, little head size, introduction to cocaine and liquor, and iodine and thyroid inadequacy are all hazard factors identified with pregnancy and birth. ADHD-related childhood diseases include respiratory infections, meningitis, encephalitis, otitis media, anemia, heart disease, thyroid disease, autism, autoimmune and metabolic disorders. Additional risk factors include brain injuries affecting the frontal lobes, toxins, medications, and dietary disorders. The relationship of dietary factors to ADHD is often problematic, especially food additives, food allergies, sucrose, gluten sensitivity and deficiency in fatty acid and iron. Maternal smoking and nicotine consumption draw the most attention in the literature, of all the environmental factors concerned, but cigarette smoking is almost always denied in practice.

Role of Adverse Home and School Environments

In a child with ADHD, adverse home environments and overcrowded classrooms may lead to and worsen the hyperactivity and inattentiveness. Those factors alone, however, are seldom the reason, and underlying hereditary or acquired causes must still be tested.

At the Pediatric Psychopharmacology Unit in Psychiatry, Massachusetts General Hospital, Boston, MA, the effect of parents with mental disorder on the behavior of children with ADHD and regular control children was examined. The prevalence of adverse family conditions, including chronic family conflict, bad family relationship, and moms with psychological disorders, was higher among 140 ADHD com-com

Clear identification of these environmental factors would result in timely action and a better outcome.

In a study of psychological disorders in families with children with ADHD, in the Department with Pediatrics, Children's Hospitals Wyler and La Rabida, University of Chicago, alcoholism, substance abuse, depression, learning difficulties and/or ADHD were more prevalent in parents with ADHD than children with control (with Down syndrome).

ADHD screening will be provided for children with a family history of mental disorders.

ADHD in Adopted Children

In an study, adoption incidence among children with hyperactive syndrome was 12 percent and more than three times the national adoption incidence in that year. For another study of ADD children a 17 percent adoption rate was registered, 8 times that seen in a standard control group or in the general population. For foster families with hyperactive adopted children, behavioral and psychological issues do not increase.

While behavioral issues are commonly believed to be more prevalent in adopted children, it must not be assumed that adverse psychological conditions exist in foster or adoptive placements. More likely reasons include an increased risk of threats to the fetus or newborn baby during unwanted pregnancies and births, and potential genetic abnormalities. Cocaine use during pregnancy and birth is commonly reported by adoptive parents of foster children in the author's ADD clinic at Children's Memorial Hospital, Chicago but is only occasionally admitted by a biological parent.

Biochemical Basis for ADHD

There is evidence that changes in brain chemistry – the neurotransmitters of catecholamine (dopamine, norepinephrine, and serotonin) – may account for hyperactivity, inattentiveness, and other ADHD symptoms; The stimulants of the central nervous system, dextroamphetamine, and methylphenidate (Ritalin R), support ADHD by increasing concentrations of catecholamine in the brain. The metabolism of catecholamine and norepinephrine levels was associated with anxiety, attention span and motor activity.

The biochemical tests are exploratory for kids with ADHD. Estimations of metabolites, or corruption items, urinary dopamine and norepinephrine or blood proteins are not of commonsense importance in the finding and treatment of ADHD, yet improve our insight into ADHD's neurobiology.

Infectious Causes of ADHD

Viral infections are related to an increased risk of ADHD during pregnancy, at birth and in early childhood. In a case-controlled study in Italy the prevalence of measles, varicella, or rubella is substantially higher in children's mothers who developed ADHD than in controls. Certain viral diseases associated with elevated ADHD prevalence and learning disabilities include HIV, enterovirus and encephalitis of the varicella zoster. Febrile seizures, frequently associated with infection with human herpesvirus in the United States and influenza A in Asia, are a risk factor for developing ADHD. Confirmation is needed of a potential association between ADHD and streptococcal infection, and a causative role for otitis media.

Perinatal and Early-Life Risk Factors

The positions of premature birth and perinatal hypoxicischemic encephalopathy in ADHD pathophysiology have been studied globally by different centres. Up to one-third of premature babies with birth weights of < 1500 g had ADHD by 5–7 years of age at the John F Kennedy Institute, Glostrup, Denmark. Birth history saw in Iceland by 196 kids with ADHD demonstrated a measurably significant expanded hazard related with low birth weight, youthful maternal age and cesarean conveyance.

Advances in NICU nursing care and improved levels of survival among premature babies have resulted in increased consideration of perinatal risk factors for ADHD. In comparison, a case-control study at the Mayo Clinic showed that pregnancy and delivery, low birth weight and twin birth were not associated with ADHD whereas positive risk factors were male gender and low rates of parental education.

Postnatal Risk Factors

ADHD is considered to be correlated with brain damage, meningitis, encephalitis, metabolic and endocrine disorders, in particular thyroid disease, contaminants and medications, and dietary deficiencies, additives and food sensitivities. A hereditary factor and acquired inclination are probably going to be essential drivers, and ecological components are likely auxiliary and fill in as triggers. Hypoglycemia, calcium, zinc, and iodine lacks are other conceivably preventable ecological reasons for ADHD.

Head Injury Causing ADHD and Learning Difficulties

For young children, head injury, however mild for degree, requires monitoring and follow-up for potential behavioral and cognitive impairments. In a sample of 95 children aged 5–15 years followed at Johns Hopkins University, Baltimore, hyperactive activity was specifically associated with the severity of the head injury. In children with previous chronic health issues and those who suffered lower extremity injuries in addition to head injury, the risk of functional disabilities following injury was increased.

Mild head injury, which is not severe to warrant hospital treatment for observation, can lead to cognitive disabilities and decreased reading and school performance in young children. Compared with a control group of pre-school children with minor injury not affecting the brain, 78 head-injured pre-schoolers screened for visual perception issues and increased incidence of dyslexia at one year after injury. The development of the visual skills needed for reading was disrupted by a mild injury to the eye.

In a 17-year-old boy who had suffered a right hemisphere injury in childhood, arithmetic and spelling skills have been affected. Work using a functional MRI at the University of Maryland, Baltimore, showed left hemisphere activation while the patient was doing arithmetic calculations. Following the injury, visuospatial abilities usually sub-served by the right hemisphere had been shifted to the left hemisphere, creating a "crowding effect" and excessive loss in mathematics and reading compared to language growth.

Low-birth-weight children at Columbia University and New York State Psychiatric Institute, with neonatal cranial ultrasound anomalies indicative of white matter injury, were at increased risk of neuro-psychiatric disorders, particularly ADHD, by the age of 6. Early-age brain injury may contribute to a reorganization of the brain positions where focus, language, and cognitive function are expressed.

Hypoglycemia and ADHD

Hypoglycemia in a baby, if unrecognized and untreated, can cause seizures and cerebrum harm that later may bring about mental impediment or learning issue and ADHD. In babies with birth anoxia or different kinds of perinatal pressure, or in neonates destined to moms with diabetes or toxemia, transient hypoglycemia may create.

Beginning stage of youth diabetes before age 5 is often exacerbated by scenes of outrageous hypoglycemia prompting moderate subjective impedance, while late beginning diabetes after age 5 and incidental scenes of extreme hypoglycemia have no impact on psychological capacity, as indicated by an investigation led in 28 diabetic kids at Trondheim University Hospital, Norway.

Transient reactive hypoglycemia can be associated with behavioral symptoms seen in ADHD following a diet with a high sugar content. A rapid increase in blood glucose can result in increased insulin secretion, with potential symptoms of hypoglycemia.

The Impact of Sugar and Other Dietary Factors in ADHD

Families also note a worsening in hyperactivity and distractivity after the child with ADHD has had a high meal with carbohydrates or a lot in candies. Although most scientifically monitored studies have failed to demonstrate major adverse effects, isolated findings appear to support conclusions of the parents.

In an investigation at Yale University School of Medicine, New Haven, CT, a 3–5-hour decline in blood glucose joined by indications of hypoglycemia (instability, heaving, weariness, and tachycardia) in kids however not grown-ups. The receptive bringing down of blood glucose had initiated an expansion in plasma epinephrine, twice as high in youngsters as in grown-ups, which was adequate to cause hypoglycemic indications. At the point when blood glucose was brought down underneath 75 mg/dl in kids, a trial of intellectual capacity utilizing evoked possibilities was significantly diminished, yet was kept up in grown-ups until the sum dropped to 54 mg/dl.

Kids are more defenseless than grown-ups to the effect of hypoglycemia on psychological capacity. An analysis of abundance admission of sugar and receptive hypoglycemia as a reason for ADHD might be made when the youngster frequently experiences progressively regular indications, including anxiety, tremor, trembling, wooziness or palpitations.

The impacts of glucose, sucrose, saccharin, and aspartame on animosity and engine movement in 30 young men, matured 2–6 years, were estimated at the Child Psychiatry Division and Developmental Psychology Laboratory, NIMH, Bethesda, MD. Eighteen young men were distinguished on parent polls as "sugar responders" and twelve were "non-responders." In a randomized, twofold visually impaired investigation, single-portion difficulties with sugar or sugar made no considerable contrasts in hostility or action rates, as surveyed by teacher and parent appraisals. In the presumed sugar responders, the standard time of hostility was related with the day by day absolute sugar consumption, yet intense sugar stacking didn't build animosity or conduct in preschool youngsters.

In an investigation of hyperactive young men with ADD and age-coordinated control subjects, the impact of a sucrose challenge on rough movement and consideration was analyzed at the Schneider Children's Hospital, New York. Hostility was not changed, yet following ingestion of sugar in the ADHD populace, absentmindedness evaluated by a consistent presentation task expanded. Conners CK at the National Children's Hospital, Washington, DC, expresses that social impacts of sugar can be appeared in youngsters with ADHD if a high starch breakfast addresses the sucrose difficulty. On the off chance that the kid has a protein supper previously or with ingestion of sugar, the impacts are turned around or blocked.

An audit of 16 existing exploration on the impacts of sucrose on the activities and perception of youngsters with ADHD, performed at Vanderbilt University, Nashville, TN, didn't show a significant unfriendly impact in the populace overall, albeit a minor impact couldn't be precluded in certain arrangements of ADHD kids. Aspartame (Nutrasweet R) utilized as a control in these investigations was considered to have no unfavorable effect on activities or cognizance, yet further investigation of aspartame wellbeing might be recommended. A few specialists have demonstrated an irritation of EEG seizure releases and headache cerebral pains following aspartame ingestion.

Feingold Food Additive Theory As aACause of ADHD

Regulated additive-free trials, Feingold diet, except in an occasional pre-school boy, have failed to show a major benefit in children with ADHD. Some parents also assume, however, that their children are susceptible to foods that contain artificial colours, flavoring agents, and preservatives. Apples, lunch foods, burgers, hot dogs, candy, dumplings, cake mixes, oleomargarine, and ice cream are avoided. The feingold diet also prohibits flavored cold beverages, soft pop, and aspirin-containing medicines.

Logical boards, set up to inquire about the eating routine's viability and supported by the FDA, have addressed treatment and hypothesis for absence of controls and measurable legitimacy. Various investigations have followed on the effect of nourishment added substances on conduct, including difficulties that incorporate added substances. In transient preliminaries, little subgroups of more youthful kids were found to react antagonistically to shading added substances yet the general advantages announced for the Feingold diet were not validated.

Determining the evidence of food additive toxicity and connection to hyperactive behavior is difficult-cult. Questionnaires performed by parents, teachers, and counselors may be biased, pro or against, and may not discuss the additive-free diet-sensitive behavioral symptoms. Belief in the Feingold theory and nutritional treatment of ADHD has diminished in the United States but waxes in

Europe and Australia, where work on the use of elimination and hypoallergenic diets for the treatment of a number of neurobehavioral conditions in children continues.

The behavioral trends associated with ingestion of azodye food colors (tartrazine and carmoisine) in a small, double-blind, monitored study at the Royal Children's Hospital in Victoria, Australia were irritability, restlessness, and sleep disruption rather than attention deficit. The author concluded that questionnaires for behavioral ratings not including sleep patterns that fail to recognize different reactors to food additives.

Role of Food Allergy in ADHD

Food allergy is proposed as a possible cause for developing ADHD. For certain prone patients hyperactive behavior has been caused by chocolate, cow milk, egg, fruit, wheat, nuts, and cheese. The Universitatskinderklinik, Munchen, Germany and the Great Ormond Street Hospital, London, played out a hyposensitization test with intradermal infusion of nourishment allergens (EPD) in 40 youngsters with ADHD. Of 20 children receiving EPD injections, they no longer responded to foods causing hyperactivity compared to 4 out of 20 receiving placebo shots. In reality, a hypoallergenic, elimination diet was rarely used, with variable outcomes. The job of nourishment excessive touchiness as a reason for ADHD is difficult to record, nervous system specialist, allergist and dietician co-activity is significant. The hypoallergenic diet requires extra research.

Iron Deficiency and ADHD

Researchers in Paris, France are documenting signs of iron deficiency in ADHD infants. Serum ferritin levels in 84 per cent of children with ADHD vs 18 per cent of non-ADHD control children were < 30 ng / ml; 32 per cent had control levels < 15 ng / ml vs 3 per cent. On additional iron, the authors record changes in focus and behavior.

Their exploration in Chicago, then again, shows that a mean serum ferritin level of 39.9 ± 40.6 ng/ml in ADHD youngsters is the same than that of sans adhd control kids, yet 18 percent of ADHD kids have rates beneath 20 ng/ml that are viewed as anomalous. None had side effects of paleness because of iron insufficiency.

A comparison of the clinical characteristics of children with the lowest levels of serum ferritin (< 20 ng / ml) with those with the highest levels of serum ferritin (> 60 ng / ml) indicates no significant difference in intensity or frequency of ADHD and comorbid symptoms or medication response. An unregulated iron supplement trial was unsuccessful and did not include a drug substitute for ADHD treatment. In our patient population a causative effect for low serum ferritin levels in ADHD has not been verified. The variance in response to iron supplements can be explained by variations in mean iron storage levels in the French and Chicago based studies. Additional regulated iron supplement trials may be suggested. Routine serum ferritin levels can be justifiable in children with ADHD.

Role of Zinc in ADHD

Many controlled trials indicate a deficiency of zinc in patients with ADHD and a beneficial response to zinc sulfate supplements, particularly in Turkey and Iran, countries with a reported endemic zinc deficiency. For another study, low levels of serum zinc were associated with inattention but not hyperactivity / impulsiveness. Some researchers are suggesting zinc sulfate supplements as adjunctive methylphenidate therapy. In the United States, there is potentially no warranty for normal serum zinc levels in children with ADHD.

Iodine Deficiency, Thyroid Function and ADHD

In certain conditions, Iodine deficiency and hypothyroidism are prenatal and posnatal risk factors for ADHD. Optimal consumption of iodine is essential to normal thyroid function and to the prevention of learning disorders and academic under-realization. In the United States, iodine is available in adequate amounts in the eating routine however iodine inadequacy is a typical event in immature nations. According to figures, 200 million people are affected by iodine deficiency diseases and 800 million are at risk globally, a total of 1 billion at risk of brain loss or malfunction. A prospective study of the neuropsychological production of offspring of women from an area deficient in iodine in Italy found ADHD in 69 per cent; no cases of ADHD were identified in an area appropriate for iodine. At early labor, the mothers were hypothyroxinemic, which led to a decrease in triiodothyronine available to the developing fetal brain. The most severe complication of the iodine deficiency is hereditary cretinism (congenital hypothyroidism). In later childhood milder types of iodine deficiency can lead to diminished cognitive function and learning disabilities. Iodine deficiency, a major international public health issue affecting underdeveloped countries in particular, can be avoided by the dietary iodine salt.

Continuous performance tests, measures of the capacity to maintain focus, were used at the University of Groningen, The Netherlands, to study 48 children with early diagnosed congenital hypothyroidism and 35 healthy controls. Sustained concentration impairments were associated with low rates of thyroid hormone pretreatment but not with the onset of treatment for hypothyroidism. Declines in performance of the sustained-attention task were attributed to cognitive, motor and motivational deficits.

At the Sanjay Gandhi Postgraduate Institute of Medical Sciences, Lucknow, India, 100 young men with delayed iodine inadequacy, not experiencing cretinism and chose for their capacity to peruse and compose were moderate students and had harmed chances to accomplish.

Iodine deficiency which does not lead to cretinism may lead to learning difficulties and poor academic motivation.

Dysfunctional thyroid. Cognition, attention, and behavioral impairments that occur with hypo- or hyper-thyroidism; Thyrotoxicosis and ADHD case reports are uncommon, and symptoms can be vague, resulting in a missed diagnosis. Treatment in 3 patients with no stereotypical symptoms of hyperthyroidism resulted in hyper-activity regulation, decreased attention span and enhanced language function. In the ADHD neurology unit at Children's Memorial Hospital, Chicago, we have observed four cases of hyperthyroidism in one year, two of goiter, using routine thyroid screening.

ADHD is recognized in patients with summed up thyroid hormone opposition (GRTH), an illness brought about by thyroid receptor quality B transformations. GRTH is portrayed by decreased reaction to thy-roid hormone by the fringe and pituitary tissues. 70 percent of influenced youngsters meet the prerequisites for ADHD in families with a past filled with GRTH announced at the National Institutes of Health, Bethesda, MD; the pervasiveness of ADHD in GRTH patients was 46 percent in another report. Given a few discoveries of an absence of relationship among's GRTH and ADHD, screening is suggested for patients with a family ancestry of thyroid brokenness.

Lead Exposure as a Cause of ADHD

Medical reports indicate that children exposed to lead may be distractible and hyperactive but few studies have used longitudinal measures to investigate the impact of lead on behaviour. A "behavioral fingerprint" trait correlated with the exposure to lead has not been established. There is often lack of evidence of cause and effect, particularly for conditions such as chronic developmental disorder and difficulties with speech articulation.

While the study is uncertain, cognitive deficiencies have associated with levels of 10 mcg / dl or higher in blood lead. In children with learning and behavioral disabilities, questions about the risk of lead exposure at home, school, or playground are significant. Determinations of pre-school blood lead are compulsory in some communities but testing in children diagnosed with ADHD and living in high-risk environments is sufficient.

A analysis of low level lead exposure and effects on intelligence, which started in 1979, was followed into the context of primary school age at the Department of Community Medicine, University of Adelaide, Australia. The IQ was contrarily identified with antenatal and postnatal blood lead focuses in 494 children, matured 7 years, from a lead purifying society, likewise at 10 mcg/dl levels. An ascent in blood lead from 10 to 30 mcg/dl, individually, activated shortfalls in verbal IQ and 6 and 5 point full scale IQ.

Three longitudinal investigations in various areas (Australia, Boston, and Cincinnati) have indicated that the decreased insight related with lead is persevering across social orders, racial and ethnic gatherings, and social and financial levels. The outcome isn't constrained to kids with social and financial detriments.

Cocaine-exposed children at risk of ADHD Cocaine-exposed babies need diligent follow-up for early detection and treatment of symptoms of neurobehaviors. A history of exposure to prenatal cocaine is normal in foster kids with ADHD who visit our ADD clinic. Presumed but not confirmed cause and effect.

A study of 30 preterm cocaine-exposed babies compared with normal controls at the University of Miami School of Medicine, FL, showed a smaller head circumference at birth, and a higher frequency of cerebral hemorrhage, disturbed sleep, nervous agitation, and tremor. The signs of abnormal brain growth and excitation were associated with elevated levels of norepinephrine and dopamine in urine, neurotransmitter chemicals essential to the ADHD cycle among cocaine-exposed adolescents. Hormonal changes have also been observed in newborns exposed to cocaine, with higher cortisol levels and lower plasma insulin levels.

Cranial ultrasonic testing of 134 exposed cocaine relative to 132 control newborns at the University of Florida, Gainesville, FL, showed an increased incidence of brain cysts and enlarged ventricles, possibly associated with cocaine-related effects on brain growth.

In 20 infants with prenatal exposure to cocaine, alcohol, marijuana, and nicotine cigarettes, increased muscle tone and motor activity, jerky movements, shakes, tremors, and back arching were observed at Women and Infants Hospital, Brown University School of Medicine, Providence, RI. In the 17 infants without cocaine exposed to alcohol, tobacco, and nicotine, or in the 20 drug-free babies, signs were observed

Dose-related effects of cocaine on neuro-behavior in exposed children tested at 3 weeks of age have been demonstrated at Children's Hospital, Boston, MA. Heavily exposed infants displayed reduced arousal control, and higher excitability than medium or unexposed babies.

The behavioral and developmental effects of prenatal cocaine observed in infancy are possibly precursors of ADHD in later childhood; a combination of drug consumption and inadequate nutrition is a combined risk factor for decreased child motor function and subsequent cognitive growth in children with a minority inner-city population.

Fetal Exposure to Alcohol, Marijuana, or Cigarettes and Increased Risk of ADHD

One feature of the "fetal alcohol syndrome" (FAS) is behavioral issues. Alcohol consumption during pregnancy and breast-feeding may cause delay in a child's development, and even an increased risk of brain hemorrhage.

Children were retarded in growth in a sample of 64 alcoholic families at Karolinska Institute, Stockholm, Sweden, and had more behavioral problems than controls up to age 4. Boys were more vulnerable compared to girls. Behavioral problems when both parents were alcoholics were more serious.

26 children of mothers who abused alcohol during pregnancy were diagnosed during their infancy at Sahlgren University Hospital, Goteborg, Sweden, and were screened for neuropsychiatric, psychological, and social problems at age 11–14. Of the following 24 infants, 10 had ADHD, 2 had Asperger syndrome, and one had mild mental retardation and autistic spectrum disorder. The severity of the disease correlated with the degree of exposure to alcohol in utero. Children whose mothers stopped drinking alcohol by the 12th week of gestation grew normally and had no learning difficulties at school. Biological, not psycho-social, factors in children with fetal alcohol syndrome are responsible for the ADHD.

Mother smoking cigarettes or weed. A systematic review of the literature found 24 studies conducted between 1973 and 2002 concerning maternal tobacco smoking. Both studies suggested a higher risk for ADHD in offspring. Maternal cigarette smoking has been related to cognitive performance and memory impairments, academic under-realization and behavioral issues in children exposed during pregnancy.

Prenatal marijuana has been connected with oversight mistakes in cautiousness exercises in a subsequent investigation of 6-year-old kids directed at Carleton University, Ottawa, Ontario, Canada, recommending a shortage in continued core interest. Cigarette smoking, marijuana use, and liquor abundance during pregnancy may effectsly affect the conduct and consideration of the baby and youngster, yet a positive causative job in ADHD has not been set up.

Many Environmental Toxins And PCBs as Possible Causes of ADHD

Our food and water sources include environmental pollutants including PCBs (polychlorinated biphenyls), PBBs (polybrominated biphenyls), nitrates, DDT, dioxin, mercury, and lead. Since the 1970s there has been no development of DDT and other pesticides including dioxin and PCBs. Despite the ban on the manufacture of such chemicals, the water of rivers and freshwater lakes also contains toxic concentrations.

PCBs were discarded years ago from electrical transformer, condenser and plasticizer factories as waste materials. Hazardous waste contaminants pollute the water from the soil at the bottom of the harbors, and are consumed by small organisms and fish. Chemicals are transmitted from fish to birds and humans, causing numerous illnesses including cancer and problems with reproduction. Man is the ultimate user in the food chains, and is exposed to the highest levels of any environmental poison.

Although environmental control measures have greatly reduced the contamination of animal feeds and food products by spillage from PCBs, certain subgroups of the population that frequently eat fish captured in lakes and streams are still at risk of poisoning. Surveys and study of fish from the Hudson River in New York State and Lake Michigan found high levels of PCB contamination above 5 ppm.

Research designed to determine the health threat of Lake Michigan fish exposure to PCBs showed a link between the amount of fish eaten and the concentration of PCBs in the research participants 'blood and breast milk. Those consuming greater quantities of fish had substantially higher levels of PCB in their blood. Children born to women who regularly ate dis-played Lake Michigan sport fish on both verbal and quantitative tests impaired short-term memory ability. A research at Wayne State University, Detroit, MI, tested cognitive performance in 212 children who were prenatally exposed to PCBs at the age of 11 (Jacobson and Jacobson, 1996). Long-term mental disability impaired memory, concentration, and ability to read, deficiencies often observed in ADHD children.

The developmental neurotoxicity of PCBs is investigated in a study by the Institute of Environmental Studies at Urbana-Champaign,

Illinois, University of Illinois (Schantz, 1996). Studies from Yusho, Japan; Yucheng, Taiwan; Michigan; North Carolina; Oswego, NY; New Bedford, MA; Inuit in Quebec's Arctic regions; and Faroe Islanders included research. For certain research methylmercury toxicity may be an external contaminant. Children born to mothers exposed to PCBs displayed behavioral and cognitive anomalies including higher rates of aggression, lower IQ scores, lower birth weight and head circumference, memory deficiencies at 4 years and psychomotor growth delays. The effects of low-level exposure to PCBs on public health were contrasted with those of lead exposure. PCB's effect on thyroid function was either primary injury to the brain in the prenatal period, or secondary.

A study of 1022 children born in the Faroe Islands in 1986–1987 to mothers who had eaten methylmercury-polluted pilot whale meat at Odense University, Denmark, found deficits in vocabulary, attention, and memory at age 7.

Subtle changes in neuropsychological functioning triggered by exposure to these environmental toxins are proposed as possible causes of ADHD and learning delays in some cases.

Impact of Diet During Infancy in the Cause of ADHD

Diets is concentrated corresponding to grown-up ailments, for example, hypertension and respiratory failure during earliest stages. Columbia University, New York, analysts broke down the pace of weight increase and diet-subordinate enhancements in natural chemistry, physiology, and conduct of 142 preterm newborn children took care of changing admissions of protein and vitality. Quickly creating newborn children had pulses, respiratory rates, dynamic rest time, and EEG levels diminished comparative with moderate developing infants. Moves in the catecholamine balance and serotonergic synapses, like those related to ADHD, were proposed as the reason for changes in diet-related autonomic reactions and fast improvement. A factor in the etiology of ADHD might be diet and weight gain during outset.

CHAPTER FOUR

Signs and Symptoms of ADHD

Within the DSM-IV diagnosis criteria, the symptoms of ADHD are described within two primary subtypes or groups:

(1) Signs of inattentiveness and
(2) Hyperactivity-impulsivity.

The current description, as defined by the American Psychiatric Association, omits symptoms of brain dysfunction and the related visual and learning disabilities. However, identification of both symptoms and signs of ADHD is crucial, particularly when it comes to identifying the cause and treatment.

ADHD as specified by DSM-IV never exists by itself. Some neuropsychiatric conditions often exacerbate the ADHD diagnosis and also change the treatment. Many of these conditions are neurological, including headache, hallucinations, tics or Tourette syndrome, and muscle control and speech and language difficulties. Others are medical or neuropsychological in nature, primarily disorder of opposition defiance (ODD), disorder of behavior (CD), and disorders of learning.

The differential diagnosis, or diseases that can interfere with any of the ADHD symptoms, includes bipolar disorders (depression, dysthymia), chronic developmental disorders (autism, Asperger's syndrome), and personality disorders (obsessive compulsive disorder (OCD), and mental retardation syndromes.

The physician who treats children with ADHD must be familiar with the related conditions and may include testing and advanced intervention methods.

Occasional "Inattentiveness" or an "Attention Deficit Disorder"?

Most children have "day dreaming" periods in school where the mind wanders transiently, but not enough to hinder learning. Inattention is an attention deficit condition (ADD) when the infant becomes incapable of maintaining focus and is frequently disturbed by external stimuli. The child must ignore or block out irrelevant distracting stimuli in order to attend. In the classroom environment, the child with ADD fails to inhibit the background "noise" Symptoms of ADD may include a lack of attention, forgetfulness, organizational failure and the inability to complete a task.

If the inattentiveness is episodic and the child is distressed, an electroencephalogram (EEG) is suggested and the risk of absence or partial complex seizures is considered. In deciding medical treatment, the difference between a persistent inattentiveness, the characteristic of ADD, and seizures is important. Stimulant medication prescribed for ADD can exacerbate inattention episodes linked to a seizure disorder. For children with ADD, and an irregular EEG, a non-stimulant drug is often preferred.

Measurement of Attention

Attention interventions include direct child observation, or indirect parent and teacher interrogation. Direct attention assessments are of three types:

(1) Alpha rhythm tracking on EEG and evoked potentials (EP);
(2) Reaction time testing, continuous performance testing, combined learning and memorization testing; and
(3) Psychometric testing such as WISC, Stanford-Binet, Detroit and Reading performance. Measures 1 and 2 are mainly applicable to research and have limited application in clinical practice. The EEG alpha activity (8–13 Hz) represents a state of relaxation and environmental inattention; the beta activity (14–25 Hz) is triggered by emotional and cognitive processes.

The EEG's computerized quantitative analysis, conducted in 25 boys with ADHD compared to 27 matched controls, showed a decline in beta and a rise in theta activity (4–7Hz). Differences in ADHD subjects were enhanced during reading and drawing tasks, especially in frontal areas of the brain. Increases in P300 wave latency, an evoked response that is produced by attention, correlate with cognitive impairment.

After stimulant therapy the response time was used to show attentiveness and cognitive development. Divided attention to multiple stimuli was controlled by induction, using operant conditioning to study visual inattention in parietal lobe-damaged subjects. The Continuous Performance Test (CPT), using commission or omission errors as inattention steps to alter stimuli and impulsiveness, is nuanced and helps certain kids to compensate for an AD. The paired associate learning (PAL) test, using WISC's coding or digit symbol subtest, is sensitive to the learning-disabled child's inattention and distractiveness with ADHD, as are regular memory assessments.

Learning requires concentration, and inattention is prone to psychometric tests of cognitive function. WISC intelligence subtest analysis – arithmetic, digital duration, and coding – shows relatively low scores in hyperactive adolescents, showing the detrimental effects of inattention and distractiveness on learning. Attention deficiency interferes with many additional intelligence and short-term memory tests performed: Stroop Color and Word Test, Stanford-Binet Comprehension Scale, Detroit Learning Aptitudes Test, and MacGinitie Reading Test. Neuropsychological testing is a significant piece of the kid's ADHD examination.

The Conners questionnaire (1969) is the most widely used early measure of attention deficit in children with ADHD. The questionnaires for the parents and teachers are either short or long. Typically they use a 4-point rating scale, and they discern hyperactivity, inattention, impulsivity, and peer interaction factors.

When Is Hyperactivity Abnormal?

Children usually often experience an excessive degree of motor restlessness, particularly in emotionally charged environments. Hyperactive behaviour is anomalous when followed by a short span of attention and distractibility, and when it is purposeless, excessive and undirected towards a clear, concrete goal. The hyperactive school-age child's trademark is the inability to concentrate and execute organized tasks. The hyperactivity level and path are anomalous, not necessarily the total daily activity. Sometimes, hyperactivity is followed by impulsiveness, a propensity to disturb others, and inability to wait in line.

In infancy the child with ADHD sometimes gets restless. As a boy, "he's in everything," and for his own safety and that of household breakables, he has to be constantly monitored. He is always fidgeting in later childhood, always "on the go," and is incapable of sitting still at dinner table. The teacher often notes an inability to sit still at school; he gets up in the classroom and runs around, speaks loudly, delays and appears to annoy and disrupt others. The hyperactivity of the motor is often followed by "visual hyperactivity," and sometimes a flight of ideas, without concentrating on the conversation topic.

Two types are distinguished in anatomical studies of the root of hyperactivity:

(1) Over-reactivity triggered by frontal lobe damage and response to external ambient-mental stimulation; and

(2) Critical over-activity caused by striatal lesions and a release of motor activity normally regulated by frontal striatal connections in the brain.

We can assume that some children with ADHD are over-reactive only when activated by a noisy environment, while others show a persistent non-environmentally based motor activity that is uninhibited. In the playground the hyperactivity may appear normal but in the classroom it may be abnormal and inappropriate.

Devices Used to Measure Motor Activity

Experimentally, several techniques were employed to assess the degree of motor activity. Which include the pedometer for quantifying gross locomotive operation; a stabilimetric cushion for measuring the degree of wiggling or fidgeting; and a grid-marked floor for assessing the time spent in one task or the degree of movement from one room to another. The author has used a system called a "actometer," an automatically revolving calendar wrist-watch with the pendulum directly attached to the wrists, so that arms or leg movements can be registered in minutes and hours. For several early controlled trials the actometer was used to treat ADHD through the use of methylphenidate. A "actometer "- like device called a" actigraph "is now available, a wristwatch-sized recorder worn on a belt.

More recently, an infrared video and motion analysis system was used during a continuous performance task (CPT) to monitor movement patterns of boys with ADHD and normal controls. Compared to controls, ADHD subjects shifted their extremities and head more than twice as much, covering a threefold greater distance and a fourfold larger area. Whole body movements were 3–4 times frequenter as well. CPT responses were more sluggish and variable. The ADHD children's behavior patterns associated with the teacher hyperactivity and inattention scores.

Such objective motor activity measures are of interest in experimental circumstances, particularly in new medical treatment trials. They can also be suggested for evidence of over-activity diagnosis where there is disparity between parent and teacher experiences. From a practical standpoint they are of minimal use in the day-to-day care of the child with ADHD.

"Subtle" or "Soft" Neurological Signs

Sometimes, slight or noticeable neurological disorders are considered "soft" symptoms. Many ADHD children are described as clumsy, or uncoordinated. They can be poor at sports, especially basketball and activities that require a fast reaction and easy movements. Soft signs are usually indicative of nervous system immaturity or delayed growth. The clumsiness and symptoms will also continue into adult life. Unlike cerebral palsy, motion incoordination is not associated with apparent weakness or spasticity in the body. Movements (synkinetic or mirror) that are typically impaired by the age of 5–7 occur in older age groups, and synchronization abilities (hopping and tandem gait) generally mastered by five years are delayed; The tempo, overflow, and rhythm of movement are essential traits of subtle neurological disorders in eliciting motor function. Timed repeated tapping of the finger, foot-to-hand overload in the tandem gait, and inability to sustain a consistent pattern of motor activity are examples used in quantitative testing of subtle sign evaluation.

Impersistence of engines is a typical soft neurological symptom of ADHD. The term was first coined to explain the challenge of sustaining a motor activity encountered by brain-injured people, while having no trouble initiating or executing the movements. The injury was located in the right brain hemisphere, especially the frontal lobe, an area that is often involved in ADHD. Motor impersistence is characterized by an inability to maintain gestures such as the following on request: "close your eyes," "look at my nose or ear," "put your tongue out" or "stretch your arms out." Besides motor impersistence, the child with ADHD is displaying an inability to suppress responses. If asked a child would not be able to look away from a stimulus. He will frequently initiate other movements such as walking when asked to hold the arms out and stand still. The instructor would say, "He can not hold his hands to himself." If he sees a pencil or a pair of scissors, he can not look at the object without putting it to its intended use, a sign of "using behaviour." Deficits in reaction inhibition are a result of inattention, a propensity to respond to distracting stimuli, and impulsiveness.

Dyspraxia, or apraxia, is another widely known soft neurological symptom associated with ADHD. Dyspraxia, given normal muscle strength, is a lack or delayed development of flexibility in purposeful activities, such as jumping, tandem walking, or scissor use. Often, the word dyspraxia refers to an inability to protrude the tongue on command, but the action is done unconsciously. One cause of apraxia can be a pause in expression. A constructional apraxia is an inability to build blocks or simply duplicate designs. Dyspraxia is caused by a dysfunction or damage to the brain's front lobes.

Dysdiadochokinesia is the neurological term for clumsiness in executing rapidly alternating forearm movements (pronation and supination). Children aged 5–7 should be able to mimic the gestures of the interviewer with-out mirroring the gesture in the opposite forearm. Involuntary manipulation of the mirror is called synkinesia, which is a typical symptom of mild brain dysfunction in ADHD. Typically, when the child is older, he will inhibit certain mirror movements.

Ataxia and incoordination may reflect an immaturity or damage to the cerebellum and its connections, often represented as clumsiness. An effort to walk a straight line is rendered unstable, and the upper limb's finger-to-nose motions trigger a tremor.

Choreiform gestures are repetitive jerky motions, usually seen by asking the child to stretch his arms. Prechtl and Stemmer (1962) identified choreiform movements, an earlier term for ADHD, as a sign of limited brain dysfunction. Choreiform gestures are rare in my experience, and not a hallmark sign associated with ADHD. These are not to be seen as "soft" signals.

A common finding with ADHD is graphanesthesia, an inability to identify numerals traceable on the skin of the palms or back. This is representative of brain parietal lobe dysfunction.

Other often elicited neurological symptoms include a propensity to walk on the toes due to tight heel cords or contractures of the Achilles tendons, and Babinski symptoms, an expansion of the broad toe and fanning from the second to the fifth toes when the foot's plantar surface is stroked with a blunt object. Under the word "soft" neurological disorders, these symptoms are not included, because they usually remain and may be indicative of permanent dysfunction of the pyramidal tracts and motor cerebrospinal system.

In a study at the Wyler Children's Hospital, University of Chicago, IL, soft neurological indicators were of predictive importance for learning disorders in preschool children aged 3–5 years. A higher neurological test score at age five was associated with a lower full-scale IQ at age seven. Neurological soft signs correctly described nearly all of the children who needed special educational assistance. In a study at Northwestern University Medical School, Chicago, irregular neurological signs similar to those found in the above test battery were previously associated with hyperactive activity, ADHD and a beneficial reaction to stimulant medication.

In a study at the Johns Hopkins University School of Medicine, Baltimore, MD, gender differences in age-related improvements in subtle motor signs was reported in 132 children with ADHD and 136 normal controls. Timed activities (e.g. finger taping) with age were improved by both controls and ADHD classes, while ADHD children were significantly slower across the age range of 7–14 years. Whereas ADHD controls and girls showed steady age-related reduction in foot-to-hand overflow and dysrhythmia (failure to maintain a steady rhythm), boys with ADHD showed no change in these signs through 14 years of age. Such variations in the "soft" pattern findings of neurological signs in brain neuroimaging research, where abnormalities in motor function areas are more common in boys than girls with ADHD. The variations in gender may have to do with earlier brain maturation in children.

In our understanding of the causes and pathological abnormalities in the brain that may clarify the mechanism of ADHD, careful examination and documentation of neurological symptoms helps. Neurological history and test results assess the need for special diagnostic laboratory examinations, such as EEG and MRI.

Developmental Coordination Disorder Diagnostic Criteria

Incoordination is a common abnormality triggered by the child with ADHD being tested neurologically. Coordination disorders are known as Developmental Coordination Disorder (200.80), or DCD, in the Diagnostic and Statistical Manual of Mental Disorders: DSM-IV definition (1994). The diagnostic DCD parameters are summed up as follows:

A. Delays in reaching motor goals, clumsiness, poor results in sports, or bad handwriting

B. Incoordination interferes greatly with the academic achievement or everyday life behaviors.

C. The disease is not caused by brain paralysis, muscular dystrophy, or any other medical condition and does not meet the requirements for a chronic developmental disorder.

Under the terms Minimal Brain Dysfunction (Clements, 1966) and DAMP syndrome, the association of coordination problems with ADHD and particularly with hyperactive behavior is identified. Minimal brain dysfunction (MBD) was a term used to identify children of near or above average intelligence, of cognitive and/or behavioral differences correlated with slight CNS functional deviations. MBD's interpretation included deficits in coordination, vision, conceptualisation, vocabulary, attention memory and control, and impulse or motor activity. The Scandinavian syndrome DAMP involves attention deficits, motor coordination and vision. The words MBD and DAMP include patients with ADHD, DCD and learning disorders, while ADHD is a symptom based condition that fails to understand the often related balance and perceptual impairment.

Relation Between Motor Performance and ADHD

In a study at the National Taiwan University of 42 school-aged children with ADHD, the performance in fine and gross motor skills was significantly impaired, as measured by the Bruininks-Oseretsky Motor Competence Test and contrasted with 42 age- and sex-matched children without ADHD. Sustained concentration and regulation of impulses are significant predictors of both fine and gross motor abilities. Hyperactivity is a predictor of gross motor incoordination but does not contribute substantially to fine motor skills. Based on the prevalence of subtle neurological symptoms in children with ADHD and impaired motor performance, a primary motor impairment is a more likely explanation to impaired concentration and loss of impulse (inhibitory) regulation than secondary motor incoordination.

Such findings suggest that the medical criteria for ADHD will include tests of motor function. Maybe a subtype of ADH and Incoordination Disorder (ADHID) will be ideal for the next version of DSM criteria.

Diagnosis and Laboratory Tests for ADHD

ADHD diagnosis is determined by reviewing feedback from parents and teachers, and by studying and interviewing the child in the physician's or psychologist's office. The parents and teachers will have completed questionnaires that evaluate focus, behavior, impulsiveness, academic achievement and social skills. Since ADHD symptoms are especially troubling when the child starts school, the teacher is often the first to draw attention to the issue and encourage the parents to contact their pediatrician.

The history of pregnancy, birth, and early development can show anomalies suggesting prenatal, perinatal, or postnatal disorders with etiological significance in ADHD. Examples are respiratory infection and nicotine toxicity during pregnancy, anoxia and prematurity at birth, and neonatal and infantile abuse, contaminants and infection. Family history may indicate hereditary influences in etiology or susceptibility to comorbid disorders (e.g., conduct disorder, tics, seizures, migraine headache, or learning disorders) or a propensity to heart abnormalities, which are critical in handling stimulant drugs. Reports of nursery, kindergarten, and high school successes and challenges will be assessed. The taking of history is followed by general physical and neurological examinations. Schoolteacher evaluations and any studies that the pediatrician, family practitioner, or psychologist has already recommended are reviewed. Reaction to preceding treatments is registered.

Genetic and environmental factors must be taken into consideration, and the need for additional studies will be calculated. The indications for EEG, MRI, blood analyses, chromosome studies, and neuropsychological evaluation are reviewed. Following the determination and examination of all requirements for the diagnosis of ADHD and complicated medical conditions, the pros and cons of stimulant or other forms of treatment are addressed.

Inquiries Posed of Parent in Making ADHD Diagnosis

At a pediatric or pediatric nervous system science discussion a parent ought to be set up to respond to the accompanying inquiries:

- What are your primary concerns, and when did the side effects start? Is the hyperactivity as well as carelessness present at home just as at school?

- What is the grade placement for your boy, the number of pupils in the class, the form of school and the bilingual education? Did any classes repeat themselves?

- Did the teacher recommend a consultation and have you submitted a written report or a completed questionnaire on behaviour, focus and achievement?

- During pregnancy, was the mother well or was she suffering from cancer, diabetes or trauma or was she using alcohol, tobacco or drugs? Takes thyroid hormone?

- Was birth normal or tricky? What was weight at birth? Was it premature birth? What were the birth scores for Apgar, or vital signs? Has the kid been breathing normally or had to be resuscitated? Has jaundice grown and needs treatment? How long in hospital was the baby?

- What were Early Development milestones? Has the kid walked 14 months, spoken 2 years in short phrases, pedaled 3 years in a tricycle, and understood 5 years in colours?

- Are there any history of hallucinations, fever attacks, episodic daydreaming or con-fused occurrences, headaches, sleep disorders, enuresis, head trauma, tics, ear infections, heart problems, asthma or chronic medication-requiring diseases?

- Have we tested vision and hearing? Has the amount of blood lead been tested?

- Does your kid have whatever other conduct gives that frequently make ADHD increasingly convoluted, for example, restriction obstruction or confusion?

- Do other family members have an ADHD past or underlying neuropsychiatric issues? There are siblings and what are their ages and achievements and academic placements? What is the parent's wellbeing and occupation? Has any family member a history of heart disease or thyroid disease? Is the local family welcoming or divided?

- If therapy is needed, how do the parents view the need and acceptance of medication?

Physical and Neurological Examinations

General physical examination involves measurements of head size, height and weight, vision and hearing, heart and blood pressure sounds, birthmarks and congenital abnormalities or dysmorphisms in the body. Neurological tests will screen for subtle neurological defects or soft symptoms, including gait and incoordination dyspraxies, dysdiadochokinesia, mirror gestures, motor impersistence, graphanesthesia, handwriting issues, handling, right-left disorientation, finger agnosia, dyscalculia, reading impairment, and speech and language disability. The detection of subtle neurological defects is an indicator of impaired maturation or complicating problems in visual perception and learning. Such results may affect treatment response and ADHD outcome.

Signs for an EEG in Children with ADH

An EEG may be regarded in the following circumstances:

- History of persistent "daydreaming" or episodic loss of awareness;

- Personal or family history of epilepsy as a precursor to stimulant medication that may precipitate seizures in susceptible patients;

- ADHD complicated by linguistic delay.

Signs for a MRI or CT Scan in a Child with ADHD

MRI or CT scan of the head is indicated for the following complications:

- Headaches and symptoms of elevated intracranial pressure or signs of systemic brain lesion;

- Seizures and an irregular EEG indicating focal epileptic discharge or focal slowing;

- ADHD exacerbated by language impairment and seizures;

- ADHD and learning disability combined and neurofibaneous syndromes (e.g. neurofibre syndromes).

Blood Tests Sometimes Indicated in ADHD

The American Academy of Pediatrics Clinical Practice Guideline (AAP, 2000), doesn't prescribe routine lab tests. Blood tests that are here and there accommodating in deciding the reason or contributing components to ADHD include:

- CBC to prevent anemia and iron deficiency;

- Serum ferritin, a measure of iron storage;

- Blood lead levels, especially in younger children with higher exposure risks;

- Liver function tests as a guide to treat ADHD with drugs that sometimes elevate liver enzymes;

- Thyroid profile, free of T4 and TSH, to rule out thyroid dysfunction, especially in children of short stature or with a family history of thyroid disease;

- Chromosome review, especially in children with signs of fragile X disease or developmental deficiency.

Indications for Electrocardiogram and/or Cardiac Consult

It is controversial that children with ADHD need to cardiovascular risk screening before beginning stimulant medication. The American Heart Association recommends routine electrocardiogram (ECG) pre-treatment while the American Academy of Pediatrics finds routine ECG as unnecessary. It is recommended for cardiac history and analysis, and for ECG and cardiac consultation, only if clinically indicated.

A complete cardiac screen consists of everything:

- History of congenital or other heart disease?

- The Sudden Death Family History?

- An early-coronary infarction family history?

- Pulse and blood pressure record;

- Heart murmur test;

- Get ECG.

Changed cardiac scan is the same as before, but for children with heart murmur or other heart defects the ECG is done selectively.

Conservative ECG pretreatment signs are indicated as follows:

- Heart murmur;

- High blood pressure and/or pulse irregularity;

- Early heart attack personal or family history;

- Participation in competitive sports.

ECG signs for ADHD medication during treatment:

- Report of chest pain or shortness of breath during exercise;

- Pulse or blood pressure abnormalities;

- Heart murmur;

- Use of higher doses of medication.

When an ECG is elevated or heart murmur is found, cardiac examination and echocardiogram are recommended. The decision to refer for cardiac consultation depends on the experience of the treating physician. The cardiologist can clear the patient for stimulant medicines, but the doctor in charge of treatment makes the final decision to treat or not to treat.

Policies related to Canadian education. Since Health Canada issued a statement warning against stimulants in ADHD patients with heart disease in May 2006, physicians 'evaluation and care of ADHD patients has changed following isolated cases of sudden death. After the advisory the proportion of non-cardiologists (0.2–15.1 percent) and cardiologists (54.8–68.6 percent) conducting a full cardiac test increased. The improvement in the use of a changed screen for non-cardiologists was 7.4–34.5 percent, and no rise for cardiologists (7.8–5.9 percent). A significant decline was seen in the proportion of non-cardiologists willing to prescribe stimulant medicines in children with possible or real heart problems. The post-advisory improvements in practice occurred despite the lack of research to address the actual cardiac effects of stimulant medication. Recommendations for consensus are needed to assess the need for pretreatment screening and to identify important risk factors for ADHD treatment's cardiac complications.

Tests of Research Interest Only

Parents often inquire about the measures commonly used in university center study studies. They include the positron emission tomography (PET) and SPECT, studies used to show improvements in the metabolism of glucose in the front lobes of ADHD patients. The experiments contain isotopes and are usually not recommended for children.

Brainstem auditory evoked potentials (BAEPs) or responses (BAERs) display changes that can be used as measures for ADD and ADHD subtype distinction. The cognitive impairments were also analyzed using evoked potentials and quantitative EEG analysis. These types of studies and the evaluation of the results require research-oriented laboratories.

Quantitative MRI can show volumetric changes in the brain, and functional MRI (fMRI) measures brain cell activity in different cerebral locations, value tests in investigating the cause and location of ADHD in the brain, and learning impairments.

Magneto encephalography (MEG) can be used to map sequences of brain activity during reading. MEG records the EEG currents 'magnetic effects during brain activation, which is a spatial-temporal measuring instrument.

Measurements of neurotransmitters, not epinephrine, and dopamine in blood, urine, and spinal fluid indicate differences in some ADHD patients and these are changed by methylphenidate therapy. ADHD's biochemical basis is an interesting research topic but not documented enough for use in practice.

Early Risk Factors For a Childhood Diagnosis of ADHD

The following factors may be predictive of early development of ADHD before a child reaches kindergarten:

- Family history of ADHD;

- Maternal smoking or drinking alcohol during pregnancy;

- Mother addicted to cocaine during pregnancy and neonatal period;

- Lower socio-economic status and low educational achievement of parents;

- Exposure to lead and elevated levels of blood lead in infants;

- Delayed milestones in the development of speech and language and psychomotor;

- Evidence of hyperactivity and irritability during infancy;

- Exposure to unstructured and critical discipline practices and unstable emotional climate in the home.

CHAPTER FIVE

Living with ADHD

Children with ADHD

ADHD is a full-time disorder which extends beyond bad behavior and school problems and affects all aspects of a person's life. Kids with ADHD aren't kids with issues but children with a serious problem. They have a complicated medical condition for them and those around them, and they stand out at all stages of development as distinct from peers and siblings (personal information, Dr Geoffrey Kewley, Learning Evaluation and Neurocare Centre, UK, 2007). There has been no psychological work conducted on how children feel and act with ADHD. Some kids may know they're different from others, but some may not have a highly established self-conception of what it means to behave differently from other kids. Research suggests that children perceive dichotomy when taking or not taking medicine, which is exacerbated by parents and teachers, e.g. feeling good / bad, happy / sad, playing nicely / fighting, etc. Children with ADHD have different social skills than those without ADHD; they can have tantrums and be violent towards others, and find it more difficult to make friends and keep them. As a result the parents may seek to fill the gap, which may contribute to the stresses they face. This is where teachers and other responsible adults can relieve some of the pressure at home by being compassionate, attentive and helpful to the school kid and knowing how ADHD presents itself. The above accounts suggest that routine and a stable environment are very important for managing symptoms of ADHD, as is continuity with the healthcare professionals the child sees.

As children grow up their symptoms are likely to change and expand into other areas. Of example, children with ADHD are more likely to be frequent smokers and drinkers between the ages of 11 and 16, and are more likely to have taken drugs. In terms of treatment, children may agree to avoid taking medicine at a particular point in their lives, or may move into adulthood by themselves.

Adults with ADHD

There is much less development in the professional discourse surrounding ADHD and adulthood than with children; indeed, most information about aetiology, symptoms or treatment comes from children's observations or studies.

Adults with ADHD can subsequently face greater obstacles in understanding and accepting and maintaining the disorder. About 30 and 50 percent of children with ADHD are believed to bring the condition into adulthood. Adult condition experiences may be characterized by feelings of restlessness and disinhibition close to those of adolescence. There is also a strong correlation of depression as well as drug abuse in adulthood.

Developmental changes can mean that levels of self-awareness or motivation toward a specific task can sometimes make the symptoms easier to manage – though this is not always the case. Living with ADHD as an adult may pose everyday challenges at work and at home, and may hinder the development of behaviors and routines that are often rooted in 'natural' lives. Problematic areas also rely on organisation. The understanding of encouragement and dedication to ADHD diagnosis and care. Organizing a busy work and social schedule can present a constant challenge; every chance to get used to some procedure or to enforce some regular structure can have a positive effect. Although new ideas and paths can be followed with some vigor, maintaining this initial drive can prove more of a challenge, and sometimes taking the long view of events will cause some disappointment. Close partnerships can be immensely rewarding at home, but these too require effort and hard work, and can sometimes prove difficult for both parties.

Adult treatment approaches

The treatment approaches for adults with ADHD are basically similar to those used in infancy. Nonetheless, there are some main differences which need to be addressed. Identification has been rare in the United Kingdom, and there are currently very few NHS specialist providers and only a handful that provide diagnosis or care facilities under the standardized AMHS system. Psychological care for adults with ADHD is not regularly provided and there have been few attempts to measure the effects of such treatments. Adults with ADHD are usually seen in a few specialist clinics which include both childhood-diagnosed developmental cases which adults that were not diagnosed during childhood. In certain cases people with ADHD were diagnosed and treated for symptoms and syndromes that coexisted together. Because of the elevated levels of ADHD among close family members, many have children with ADHD, and need extra assistance to provide their children with adequate support.

Medication

While the number of drug trials in adults is much lower than in children, they clearly show the effectiveness of stimulants in reducing the level of ADHD symptoms in adults who meet diagnostic criteria for ADHD. Adult treatment regimes are similar to those used in children although higher doses are used in a few cases.

While stimulants in children and adults are the most researched and the most common treatment for ADHD, their use in adults remains controversial across Europe. In the United Kingdom, treatment of ADHD in children has improved significantly over the last decade, with a marked rise over ADHD diagnoses and a doubling in stimulant prescriptions between 1998 and 2004 (NICE 2006b). This shift in viewpoint, however, is only gradually filtering through to those interested in managing the adult population. It remains an irony that many medications are not approved for use in adults but are considered safe and effective in children and young people.

Stimulants are normally the first-choice pharmacological treatment for ADHD in both adults and children. Methylphenidate and dexamfetamine are available in the United Kingdom, but still unlicensed for adult use. There is some evidence for the safety and efficacy of stimulants in children, and a growing amount of evidence for effectiveness in adults. The effects of stimulants on ADHD symptoms vary from many other medical therapies, as there is an immediate impact, beginning within 30 minutes from the initial dose and lasting for 3 to 4 hours in the case of IR preparations. Throughout the day, those preparations must be taken several times. MR precautions, which last around 8 to 12 hours and are typically only taken once a day, are especially useful for those who are forgetful or disorganized until the effects of the drug begin to wear off.

Atomoxetine is typically the second-line form of treatment for ADHD in adults.

Third-line options include bupropion, modafinil, and noradrenergic antidepressants such as imipramine, venlafaxine, and reboxetine, but there is less clear evidence for such medicines in reducing adult ADHD symptoms. Atomoxetine is available in the United States for the treatment of ADHD in children and adolescents, but it is approved in the United Kingdom only for the treatment of adolescents who began atomoxetine in childhood or adolescence.

Psychological Therapies

Psychotherapeutic approaches used to treat people with ADHD include psychoeducation, use of networks of support, testing in skills, CBT, coaching and therapy.

In adults with ADHD, therapeutic approaches using a cognitive model to teach techniques for controlling ADHD were used, typically as a supplementary therapy for the use of stimulant medication, although they may be appropriate for adults with substantial reduction of symptoms with age. Qualitative work has indicated that therapeutic care starts at the point of diagnosis, during which individuals with ADHD deal with their condition and with the effects of the illness on their lives through a cycle of adjustment. Then, psychological care can change to focus on coping with coexisting psychiatric problems, psychological problems, and ability deficits. The point is to assist individuals with creating techniques to give regular daily existence structure and improve relational aptitudes so they can work all the more effectively and accomplish their latent capacity. For sure there is a decent base of proof for clinical treatment of numerous clinical issue related with ADHD.

Many types of psychotherapy such as counseling or client-based psychotherapy have played a part in helping certain people come to terms with their personal and emotional lives and better understand how ADHD has affected them. Coaching approaches mirror a mentoring approach by helping individuals with ADHD to regularly rehearse newly acquired skills; these were used as an alternative to adult cognitive community services. Formal studies have not yet been performed on the efficacy of psychotherapy and coaching, although many adults with ADHD say that they benefit from these strategies.

Special issues for adults diagnosed with ADHD

Educational and occupational disadvantage

ADHD adults generally record a history of poor academic success and underperformance. These problems begin in years of elementary school and often go on into adolescence and young adulthood. This is a time when young people are faced with important decisions regarding their future, yet young people with ADHD are less likely to make plans compared to their peers. Most likely, learning problems are strongly associated with signs of ADHD. Person or small group tuition, additional test time (if required in a separate room), help with time management, goal setting, prioritization of tasks and study techniques, can help to reduce their effect.

Young people are expected to assume greater personal responsibility for structuring and managing their time, prioritizing activities and meeting deadlines with increasing age, further schooling and/or the workplace. This can explain why adults with ADHD frequently underdo academically in contrast with their family members 'expectations and achievements. They also deviate from family standards of employment status by being employed in considerably lower-ranking occupations than their siblings. While some people with ADHD find work that is consistent with their symptoms, others report higher job problems rates including higher job turnover and periods of unemployment. Instead of pursuing a profession, they also seek out several different forms of occupations.

Drug abuse

The clarification for raised degrees of substance use issue in individuals with ADHD is intricate. ADHD is a hazard factor for substance use issue through three potential systems:

1. Increased levels of reward- (risk-) behaviour;

2. Increased levels of psychosocial impairment (oppositional disorder and childhood disorder associated with substance abuse); and

3. Self- for symptoms of ADHD.

Disorders with extreme drug use should be handled first in most situations because of the known complications and impairments associated with such behaviour. Continuing abuse of the drug can interfere with the assessment of the reaction to ADHD treatment – associations can occur and side effects may be increased. While all substance use should be minimized before pharmacological treatment begins, it should be recognized that the persistence of ADHD symptoms may maintain misuse of the substance in order to supplement the symptoms with medication. However, self-treatment with stimulants is uncommon, whereas the use of alcohol and cannabis to dampen adult ADHD-related symptoms is far more common.

There is no proof accessible to help the feelings of dread of certain clinicians that the utilization of energizers in ADHD can add to chronic drug use either by sensitisation or as a pathway to different medications. While there might be a hazard that a few people with substance dependence issues will sell energizers, recollect that when grown-ups use energizers accurately, they are not propensity framing or addictive, and they don't trigger rapture. Also, there is proof from the subsequent research that medication misuse issues are developing.

Crime Correlation

Early onset and recurrent antisocial behavior are generally related to ADHD.

Longitudinal studies have shown that ADHD independently predicts the development of antisocial behaviour, a developmental pattern which is believed to be influenced by aspects of the family environment.

The association between ADHD and crime is increasingly recognized and regarded with concern. Studies in the US, Canada, Sweden, Germany, Finland and Norway show that about two-thirds of youth offender facilities and up to half of the adult prison population in childhood tested for ADHD positively and many tended to be symptomatic. A significant number of people may have mild symptoms and are in partial recovery from the effects of their ADHD. All these studies have shortcomings in their methodologies, yet the prevalence of young people and adults with ADHD in the prison population seems to far surpass that recorded in the general population (that is, 3–4 percent of children and 1 percent of adults).

ADHD was associated with an early onset of criminal behaviour, well before the age of 11, and high levels of recurrence were observed in institutionally incarcerated young people with ADHD. Young people are likely to experience more serious and omnipresent symptoms than older offenders housed in adult jails, and this most likely accounts for the significantly higher incidence of ADHD reported in young offender institutions. The 'revolving door' between jail and probation and the community for these young people is most likely closely correlated with the extent of their ADHD symptoms.

A meta-analysis of 20 ADHD research identified a clear correlation between ADHD interventions and criminal / delinquent behaviour, and concluded that ADHD is a factor that should be addressed in providing recovery services to offenders, beginning with early intervention programs and continuing with adult offender rehabilitation and supervision.

Differential diagnosis and mistaken diagnosis

Coexisting disorders in adulthood include personality disorder (especially antisocial and borderline disorder), bipolar disorder, obsessive-compulsive disorder and, to a lesser degree, psychotic disorder. Adults with severe mental illness such as autism or extreme learning impairment often have issues with concentration and levels of activity, yet these conditions do not occur more often in individuals with ADHD than in the normal population.

However, there is a difficulty in that care issues are common to many psychiatric disorders; therefore adults with other psychiatric problems may appear to have ADHD symptoms. On the other hand, this also indicates that there is a population of adult psychiatric patients in whom the ADHD condition has not been identified and where inadequate therapies for alternative conditions such as anxiety, depression, cyclothymia and personality disorder have been put in place. It may account for the high interaction rates reported for adults with ADHD with mental health facilities, which in turn has significant cost implications.

ADHD is often misdiagnosed in adults because the novice ADHD diagnostician has possible 'traps.'

In adulthood, ADHD does not appear in children who have more signs of hyperactivity, for example, in the same way as ADHD. The age criterion is critical for separating ADHD from the conditions of later onset and, unless care is taken to rule out the presence of the other conditions, a high rate of wrongly reported cases can occur.

Psychopathology is superimposed in two major forms for other medical disorders.

First, the repetitive feature-like features of ADHD symptoms starting in early childhood and persisting in adulthood are often mistaken for characteristics of a personality disorder. This happens in particular with personality disorders in cluster B (that is, antisocial, borderline and emotionally unstable personality disorders), as these include symptoms commonly associated with adult ADHD such as mood disturbance, impulsiveness and outbursts of anger. Second, the commonly recorded volatile and irritable mood of adults with ADHD is a symptom which overlaps with the one seen in major affective disorders. Both bipolar disorder and ADHD are characterized by changes in hyperactivity, distractiveness, inattention and mood. However, the distinction is that ADHD's mood state is irritable and unpredictable, instead of having components of euphoria and grandiosity. More recently, it has been suggested that very early 'youthful mania' is characterized by an irritability mood rather than euphoria, and by chronicity rather than fluctuation. If this change in meaning is acknowledged then this distinction from ADHD will become highly problematic in young people.

ADHD's Effect on Family Life and Relationships

ADHD can significantly affect family life and kinships (World Federation for Mental Health, 2005).Parents of children with ADHD need a lot of support to help them manage the problems they have with their child. Not only is it a case of having to cope with the daily challenges of living with a child with ADHD; parents also have to deal with school issues that are so prevalent in these children, many of which require a declaration of special educational needs. Kids with ADHD require a lot more support and guidance in most of their daily lives than their peers. It is a complete condition which needs full-time treatment. The pain and fatigue felt by many parents is something that practitioners need to recognize.

Parents are concerned about the effect that the lack of awareness of ADHD by health and social care providers, school workers and the broader public may have on their child's life:

- 91% of parents were frequently depressed or worried about their child's life

- 68% said their ADHD child was excluded from social activities due to their symptoms of ADHD

- 61 percent said their family activities were disrupted

- 51 percent said the diagnosis took too long

- 63 percent said their primary care doctor did not know much about ADHD.

According to a study conducted by the World Mental Health Federation, the average time taken to receive an assessment and eventual diagnosis is 2.44 years, with 17 percent waiting for more than 5 years (World Mental Health Federation, 2005). As the accounts above indicate, parents and caregivers should provide healthcare practitioners with a wealth of knowledge about the signs and activities of their child's ADHD, which can not only allow the specialist to make an appropriate diagnosis, but also offer treatment and care tailored to the individual needs of the child.

A variety of societal misunderstandings about ADHD need to be resolved in the best interests of children and their families. To resolve these misunderstandings, it is important to learn more about the effect of the condition on families, and specifically how well the needs of families are handled.

Families impacted by ADHD will benefit from assistance from all departments, including education, social care, their GP, mental health services and, in some cases, the criminal justice system and police. Both services can better serve families and others with ADHD by working together to give the child / young adult and family a support program. Medication alone isn't the answer; a lot of help is also needed to treat the condition. Behavioral control and moderation, organized tasks and an incentive-based compensation program may also be of value.

A kid with ADHD may have one or the two guardians presuming that the youngster is not quite the same as other kids and effectively seeking after clinical help. Often teachers are the first to identify ADHD symptoms, seek treatment, and assist parents and children alike. As the personal accounts of parents illustrate, and as the Mental Health of Children and Young People in the United Kingdom study reports in 2004, teachers 'are likely to have worried about [the child's] overactivity, impulsiveness, and insufficient attention,' which may lead to difficulties acquiring basic skills at school: 'Almost three-quarters (71%) of children with hyperkinetic conditions have suffered from hyperkinetic issues. Above all, the accounts talk of the challenges of seeking the best educational atmosphere where the child can be encouraged and grow, and where he or she can fulfill their individual needs.

Parents can also receive assistance from mental health, primary care or educational professional programs. There are also concerns as to why ADHD occurs (or whether the child is just naughty) and at what point a diagnosis should be made, which may clarify why a referral to a healthcare professional is daunting for certain parents. Parents may seek informal advice from relatives, friends, self-help organizations or the internet, this can be their only support.

Parents will inevitably face the dilemma of starting treatment for ADHD symptoms, or of using alternative therapies or changing their child's diet. If parents choose medication, they the feel guilty and agree to have 'medication vacations' in order to encourage the 'true kid' to emerge (Singh, 2005). Parents can receive mixed media messages about ADHD medication, and believe too many children are taking medication. According to Great Britain's Mental Health of Children and Young People, 'about 2 in 5 (43%) children with hyperkinetic disorder are taking some sort of medication.' Sometimes, ADHD goes hand in hand with other disorders, such as deficiency of conduct, making behavioral and emotional problems much more complex. Such problems have implications for many aspects of the lives of children and young people; it is estimated, for example, that approximately one third of children with hyperkinetic conditions are excluded from education. These children may continue to have legal issues as well.

Parents and carers of children with ADHD can find it difficult to be a mother or father, given this collection of circumstances. When compared to parents without children with ADHD, they are more likely to split if they are a couple, have emotional problems and work less well than a family.

Parents and caregivers therefore need guidance from healthcare professionals who should consider:

- Ensure that parents / caregivers have good support networks, such as access to a self-help group, and are aware of local and national organizations

- Recommend useful resources (books, newsletters, websites, etc.)

- Help parents / caregivers find places for their children to improve their self-esteem (for self-help).

- Recognizing that ADHD is a complex disorder and rarely without coexisting conditions

- Recognizing that transition and change can be difficult

- Helping parents / families to obtain support for relationship / marriage problems and any siblings

- Encourage parents to maintain a diary of behaviors to feed back into CAHMS meetings and other healthcare professionals

- Ask the parents to complete a questionnaire before beginning treatment so they can discuss variations.

CHAPTER SIX

Differentiating ADHD in Adults From Other Coexisting Conditions

Personality disorders

There is still substantial nosological uncertainty arising from the early development and severity of ADHD behavioral symptoms, which often manifest rather than signs as normal behaviors or personality characteristics. The difference in the concept of a trait and a symptom is that symptoms signify a transition from a typical pre-morbid condition, such as the onset of adult depression or insanity, while traits are assumed to be permanent. Current medical training in adult mental health continues to focus on distinguishing between signs and characteristics, resulting in a nosology that does not suit the definition of ADHD properly. First, due to the traitlike nature of ADHD symptoms, severe psychopathology frequently goes unnoticed or is considered a feature of personality, resulting in a different range of clinical course and outcome therapies and goals compared with ADHD. Secondly, since ADHD symptoms are often associated with chronic destructive and oppositional behaviour, or weak interpersonal ability growth, this is often believed to be an entrenched and therapeutically resistant set of behavioral traits. Further ambiguity emerges from the concept of personality disorders in cluster B, such as antisocial, bipolar, and emotionally dysfunctional personality disorder, which include signs such as mood disturbance, impulsivity, and outbursts of rage typically known to coexist with ADHD in adults.

The diagnostic problem is to determine whether there is evidence of ADHD, i.e. if the clinical conditions have been met in childhood and whether the symptoms of ADHD that started in childhood have continued and continue to cause severe disability. Although the diagnostic focus will be on the key symptoms that describe inattention, hyperactivity and impulsivity, it's also important to note that mood disturbance and impulsivity are often seen in adults with ADHD. Within the sense of a particular ADHD syndrome, caution must be taken to differentiate between uncontrolled, impulsive, oppositional and antisocial behaviors that occur from those that do not. Of this purpose, it is also helpful to examine particular ADHD-specific symptoms such as short attention span, inconsistent results, distractibility, forgetfulness, disorganization, physical restlessness, and over-talkativity rather than concentrating solely on the incidence of unadjusted and destructive behaviors.

Mood disorders

Depression

For adult ADHD, erratic and irritable mood is often observed, which is typically not the product of coexisting depression or bipolar disorder. The overlap of mood symptoms means care must be taken to rule out the possibility of a major affective disorder and mood labiality does not occur solely in the context of such disorders. Participating in the symptoms and psychopathology time-course can help to differentiate the two. Early onset, persistent trait-like pattern, regular mood changes during the day, no recent regression or serious exacerbation frequently accompany ADHD, whereas extreme low or high moods, continuous mood change over long periods of time and recent development are more characteristic of a primary affective disorder. A primary diagnosis of ADHD can be made for those people previously diagnosed with atypical depression, cyclothymia or dysfunctional mental personality disorder.

Bipolar disorder

The distinction between ADHD and bipolar disorder has traditionally been fairly simple to make. Bipolar disorder has been related to euphoria, grandiosity and a cycling regimen, with each episode lasting at least several days. In contrast, ADHD has been considered a persistent disability in which euphoria is not a feature in particular. The goal-directed mania over-activity is generally seen as contrasting with ADHD's disorganized and off-task activity. Individuals with ADHD often have difficulty sleeping but they complain about their lack of sleep unlike mania or hypomania and often feel exhausted during the daytime. Generally speaking, individuals with ADHD complain that they can not work efficiently, and this is often correlated with constant low self-esteem, quite different from the mania-like feelings of increased performance. In ADHD thoughts are also described all the time as 'on the go,' but unlike mania or hypomania, they are experienced as distracted, muddled and inefficient and there is no subjective sense of improved thought process performance.

However, the definition of bipolar disorder has been extended to include cases where the change in mood is not euphoria but irritability or persistent mixed affective states, and where the cyclic existence consists of multiple changes within one day (indistinguishable from a erratic, labile mood). This points to a very significant resemblance between this so-called ultradian variant of bipolar disorder and ADHD in the standard definitions. An erratic and over-reactive mood is very frequently seen in ADHD although it is not part of the diagnostic criteria, and the development of an oppositional disorder, in which frequent tantrums are normal, can be defined as a 'irritable' condition and thus leads to a bipolar diagnosis.

One of the key questions concerns the validity of a narrowly defined diagnosis definition of bipolar disorder or whether mood instability / irritability in the presence of ADHD can be represented more accurately by a new aspect, such as mood dysregulation. The classic definition of mania should be retained until the appropriate clinical evidence are available: a diagnosis of bipolar disorder includes euphoria, grandiosity and episodicity, and the distinction between ADHD and bipolar disorder remains clear.

Anxiety disorders

People with ADHD much of the time report elevated levels of rating scale nervousness. Nonetheless, an increasingly nitty gritty psychopathology enquiry shows that the ADHD disorder imitates certain parts of tension in specific cases. People with ADHD can think that its hard to manage social conditions since they can't focus on discussions; voyaging trouble since they can't design the excursion; and shopping trouble since they may get bad tempered holding up in lines and in light of the fact that they may overlook things and be profoundly scattered. Issues that the vast majority underestimate with essential day by day undertakings are a wellspring of extraordinary concern and are frequently trailed by staying away from upsetting exercises and low confidence. Such legitimate stresses and responses, related to perpetual mental action, can assume the presence of a mellow to direct condition of tension, however inadequate with regards to the clinical indications of nervousness issue. A significant differentiation is to consider whether the side effects have a comparable beginning and time course to ADHD, or whether they happen ramblingly and in light of stressors, which is nervousness trademark.

Psychotic disorders

Extreme absentmindedness may once in a while copy the idea issue indications found in certain psychoses, for example, crash, unrelated points of view, circumstantiality and trip of thoughts. Cautious checking of both insane side effects and ADHD indications is suggested, yet recognizing the lingering side effects of a significant dysfunctional behavior from the constancy of ADHD side effects can be hard.

Diagnosis

A diagnosis of ADHD should only be made by a licensed physician, pediatrist or other appropriately trained healthcare practitioner with experience and expertise in the treatment of ADHD, on the basis of:

- A full psychological and psychosocial assessment of the person; this should include consideration of actions and symptoms in the different contexts and settings of the person's daily life;

- A complete history of development and psychology, and

- Observer accounts and evaluation of the mental condition of the individual.

An ADHD diagnosis should not be made solely on the basis of assessment scale or observational results. However, assessment scales such as the Conners assessment scales and the Strengths and Difficulties questionnaire are important adjuncts, and observations (at school, for example) are useful when symptoms are in doubt.

In the diagnosis of ADHD, signs of hyperactivity / impulsiveness and/or inattention should:

- Meet the diagnostic requirements in DSM- or ICD-10 (hyperkinetic disorder), and

- Be correlated with at least mild psychological, social and/or educational or occupational disability based on interviews and/or direct observation in multiple environments, and

- Be pervasive, occurring in two or more important environments;

Require an evaluation of the needs of the individual, coexisting conditions, social, family and educational or occupational circumstances and physical health as part of the diagnostic process. There should also be an evaluation of the mental health of their parents or carers for children and young people.

ADHD should be taken into consideration in all age ranges, with symptom guidelines changed for age- behavioral changes.

Wherever practicable, parental experiences should be taken into account when assessing the clinical value of disability that results from the effects of ADHD when children and young adults.

Post-diagnostic advice for parents

Following an ADHD diagnosis, healthcare practitioners will recommend offering ADHD self-instruction manuals to all parents or carers of all children and young people, and other resources such as videos, focused on effective parenting and behavioral strategies.

CHAPTER SEVEN

Oppositional, Conduct, and Other ADHD Comorbid Disorders

Sometimes ADHD-related medical conditions include oppositional defiant disorder, behavior disorder, mood disturbances, and anxiety disorders including obsessive compulsive disorder. These are referred to as comorbid disorders. They complicate the treatment of ADHD and may require medical or psychological intervention if severe enough to affect school and social functioning. The following concepts from the DSM-IV diagnostic criteria are simplified for practical purposes.

Oppositional Defiant Disorder

The criteria for the diagnosis of oppositional defiant disorder include at least five of the following, present for at least six months:

- Loses temper often

- Argues with adults

- Refuses to do chores

- Annoys other people

- Blames others
- Easily annoyed
- Often angry
- Often spiteful
- Swears frequently

Conduct Disorder

A behavior disorder is severe if at least three of the following criteria have been in place for at least six months:

- Steals
- Runs away from home
- Lies
- Sets fires
- Plays truant
- Breaks into someone's house, building or vehicle
- Destroys other property
- Cruel to animals and/or people
- Sexually abusive
- Starts fights, with or without a weapon.

Mood Disorders

ADHD-complicating mood disorders may include manic and/or depressive spells, bipolar disorders, cyclothymia and dysthymia.

A manic episode consists of an elevated or irritable mood sufficient to impair school and social functioning and associated with at least three of the following:

- Increased self-esteem
- Sleeplessness
- Excessive talk
- Flight of ideas
- Distractibility
- Excessive goal-driven activity
- Excessive expenditure and spread buying

A depressive disorder is recognised by at least five of the following symptoms, persisting for at least two weeks, and one consisting of either depressed mood or a lack of interest in activities:

- Depressed mood
- Lack of interest in activities
- Loss or irregular weight gain
- Inability to sleep or prolonged sleepiness

- Anxious or sluggish

- Extreme exhaustion

- Remorse feelings

- Failure to think or focus

- Death or suicidal thoughts

Bipolar symptoms are psychotic, depressed or both, with frequent psychotic or depressed episodes and do not necessarily follow the complete medical requirements.

Cyclothymia is characterized by episodes over a year or longer that are hypomanic and depressed but not major, and never for more than two months at a time without certain symptoms.

Dysthymia is a depressed or irritable condition that occurs regularly, without major depression, for at least one year and that is accompanied by at least two of the following:

- Weak or excessive appetite

- Lack of or excess of sleep

- Loss of energy or exhaustion

- Poor self-esteem

- Inability to focus and concentrate

- Hopelessness

Anxiety Disorders

Panic disorder, phobias, obsessive compulsive disorder, post-traumatic stress disorder, and common anxiety disorder include anxiety disorder.

Panic disorders are characterized by shortness of breath, dizziness, rapid heart rate, shivering, sweating and pain. Prolapse of the mitral valve may be associated with these symptoms, and exposure to amphetamine or caffeine, or elevated thyroid levels, may mimic the syndrome.

Phobias include a fear of being alone in groups, in crowds, on bridges and driving alone (agoraphobia); and a fear of communicating in public or answering questions in class (social phobias). Children may be afraid to attend birthday parties, or other community functions.

Obsessive compulsive disorder consists of recurrent and persistent, irrational ideas and thoughts (obsessions), and repeated, purposeful, obsessive actions (compulsions) in response to obsessions. Compulsive behavior examples include repeated rubbing of things, and hand washing.

Post-traumatic stress disorder is an pathological response to a distressing incident, characterized by recurrent distressing memories or trauma-related hallucinations, avoidance of trauma-related events, sleep disruption, irritability, and incapacity to concentrate on school work.

Generalized anxiety disorder is an extreme degree of anxiety and concern over grades at school and social contact with peers. Symptoms include tremor, restlessness, palpitations, vomiting, dizziness, concentration problems and irritability. The signs of anxiety disorder can be mimic by caffeine addiction or excess thyroid.

Psychiatric Conditions Prevalence In children with ADHD

Children with ADHD complicated by severe mood disorders and anxiety disorders are likely primarily referred to the psychiatrist or psychologist of the child. The pediatric and pediatric neurologist also treats patients with mild to moderate oppositional defiant and conduct disorders. Estimates of incidence of comorbid conditions are based on the prescribing doctor's specialty; higher occurrence rates may be expected for children referred to psychiatric clinics and psychologists. Most clinical studies concerning ADHD children with comorbid psychological conditions were performed in departments of psychiatry at major universities and medical centres. Children treated in pediatric practice and in child neurology clinics should expect lower prevalence rates.

Relationship Between ADHD and Oppositional Defiant Disorders

Comorbid oppositional defiant disorder (ODD) with ADHD is a more severe issue than conductive disorder (CD). Most kids with ADHD do not have CDs. Many with CD develop the condition before age 12 years, and have had signs of Unusual almost always for several years beforehand.

There are various results for ODD children with CD, and those without. ADHD CD is associated with a higher prevalence of adolescent drug abuse, and a higher rate of anxiety and mood disorders.

At the Pediatric Psychiatric Service, Massachusetts General Hospital, Boston, the link between oppositional defiant disorder (ODD), conduct disorder (CD), and ADHD was evaluated:

- Of 140 children with ADHD, 65 percent had comorbid ODD and 22 percent had CD at initial examination.

- 32 per cent of ODD children had a comorbid CD.

- Children with CDs also had Chances that many years followed CD.

- Children with both ODD and CD had more serious ODD symptoms, more psychiatric disorders including more bipolar disorder, and more irregular behavioral scores compared to non-comorbid ADHD children.

Neurological soft signs associate with the presence of ODD and CD symptoms, as well as anxiety, phobias, depression or dysthymia. In a study of 56 high-risk boys aged 7–10 at the New York State Psychiatric Hospital, NY, presentation of soft signs at neurological review was a risk factor for psychiatric symptoms of childhood onset, as well as ADHD.

Variables That Predispose to Conduct Disorders in Children with ADHD

ADHD and learning disabilities lead to illnesses, but the primary cause is to be associated with severe, incoherent parenting. Studies at Queens College, Flushing, NY, and the London Institute of Psychiatry also showed a link between parent-aggressive behavior and child aggression, particularly among boys. In 10 per cent of children in an urban community, violent behavior occurred, and the majority of juvenile delinquents had behavioral problems by age 7. The NY Study correlated reduced serotonergic activity, a neurochemical process, with aggression.

Impact of an Adverse Family Environment on ADHD and Comorbid Disorders

Adverse family conditions, persistent parental tensions, and mother-influencing mental disorder affect the outcome of ADHD and treatment response. In a survey of 140 children with ADHD at Massachusetts General Hospital, Biederman and associates (1995) found elevated rates of environmental deprivation in children with ADHD relative to subject controls. Parental tension and exposure were especially prevalent in moms with mental illness. Fortunately, environmental adverse factors did not affect the risk of developing comorbid behavior disorder, depression or anxiety.

Researchers at the University of Chicago found that, in an investigation of social and developmental issue in families of young people of ADHD, children with ADHD were expected to have a parent affected by drug use, other alcohol abuse, depression, violence, academic incapacity and ADHD. ADHD screening should be provided for children with a family history in mental disorders. Psychosocial therapy is recommended for the families affected.

Childhood Conduct Disorder and Adult Criminality

Children with ADHD and behavioral problems are at greater risk of criminal activity and detention in adolescence and adult life. Severe behavioral disturbances in childhood and antisocial behavior in teenagers, when controlled by early psychosocial intervention, may be predictors of subsequent conviction for crime.

In some exploration, hyperactive youngsters are multiple times more probable than typical to create conduct issues and a resulting increment in culpability.

Mood and Anxiety Disorders Connection to ADHD

Psychiatrists also consider a link of cause and effect between ADHD symptoms and anxiety or depression (Silver, 1992). Neurologists, on the other hand, advocate an endogenous biological etiology for ADHD, and find anxiety or mood disorders to be secondary symptoms, often precipitated by medication.

A methylphenidate-induced depressive reaction occurs especially in larger doses, and in children with a genetic susceptibility to mood disorders. The mood condition may also be associated with atomoxetine (Strattera R), a non-stimulant drug.

A research at the Massachusetts General Hospital, Boston, explored a family relationship between ADHD and bipolar disorder in 140 children and their first-degree relatives who were affected. Relatives were at fivefold increased risk of bipolar disorder if the child with ADHD also suffered from bipolar disorder. The comorbid presentation of ADHD and bipolar disorder tends to be a distinct subtype of ADHD that affects mainly boys and has a high family risk of ADHD, bipolar disorder and major depression. This subtype, however, was rare, occurring in just 5 per cent of ADHD children. The findings failed to support the depression hypothesis as a cause of ADHD.

Physicians also face separation between biological and medical triggers for behavioral and mood disorders compounded by reports of hyperactivity, distractivity and impulsiveness. Recognizing early onset mood disorders should cause removal or dose reduction of stimulant or other medication and, where appropriate, referral to colleagues specialized in child psychology and psychiatry.

Teenage mania and ADHD. The Department of Psychology, University of Cincinnati, Ohio, has confirmed a correlation between teenage mania and ADHD. Of the 14 adolescent bipolar patients admitted to hospital for acute mania or hypomania treatment, 8 (57%) met the DSM criterion for ADHD diagnosis. ADHD patients had higher scores on a Mania Assessment Scale than those with only bipolar disorder.

In a 3- to 12-year sample of two groups of school-age patients treated at the Psychiatric Departments of the Universities of Pittsburgh, and California at San Diego, and Harvard University, clinical symptoms and outcome of childhood-onset dysthymic disorder were correlated with major depressive disorder. Dysthymic disorder has an older onset age than that of major depressive disorder. Symptoms of feeling unloved, irritability and frustration were similar, but feelings of guilt, poor focus, loss of appetite, insomnia and tiredness were less frequent than in major depression. Dysthymic patients increased risk of major depressive disorder and bipolar disorder.

Oppositional defiant and behavioral conditions occurred more often in a dysthymic group of children than in those with severe depression, treated as in-patients in a child psychiatry clinic at Stony Brook State University, New York.

In a study at the Pediatric Psycho-Pharmacology Unit, Massachusetts General Hospital, Boston, children with the mixed subtype of ADHD (inattentive and hyperactive-impulsive) displayed the greatest psychological impairments compared with other subtypes. Hyperactive-impulsive patients didn't benefit from controls on depression, social functioning, IQ, and academic achievement tests.

ADHD and Drug Abuse Disorders in Adolescents

Young people with ADHD had a higher danger of liquor or substance abuse issues as non-ADHD screens in a prior investigation at the Department of Psychiatry, Massachusetts General Hospital, in Boston.Substance misuse in 15 percent of 140 adolescents with ADHD and with the same incidence in 120 typical control subjects had occurred at 4-year follow-up. In puberty, ADHD itself does not predispose to substance abuse. In patients with a background marked by mental or burdensome disarranges, the danger of liquor and substance abuse was raised, yet not in those with an oppositional insubordinate confusion, extreme despondency, or nervousness. Uncomplicated by conduct issue, the oppositional insubordinate condition didn't incline to substance misuse.

Impact of Stimulant Treatment on Risk of Drug Abuse

Latest research at Massachusetts General Hospital investigated the impact of early stimulant therapy for ADHD in adolescent boys and girls on the resulting incidence of substance use disorders (SUDs) and cigarette smoking. Stimulant-exposed adolescents with ADHD were 73 per cent less likely than non-exposed ones to be diagnosed with SUD. The childhood stimulant therapy for ADHD has a major protective effect on the development of any adolescent SUD and cigarette smoking (P=0.001). Late stimulant therapy doesn't affect the risk of drug misuse or drug dependency.

These findings will relieve the common worry of parents whose children are prescribed stimulant medications for ADHD.

Adult ADHD and Substance Misuse Relative to Teenagers

Studies suggest adults with ADHD are more vulnerable than teens to substance abuse. A rapid increase in substance abuse can be expected in adolescent ADHD subjects as they become adults, especially if they have not received treatment for ADHD beforehand.

At the Veteran's Affairs Medical Center, West Haven, CT, Comorbid ADHD and drug abuse were studied in adolescents and adults. Drug use and abuse were linked to attempts to self-medicate ADHD symptoms, particularly in previously untreated adolescents. ADHD prescribed medical care was found to decrease the appetite of drugs in adults with comorbid ADHD and substance abuse, and to increase function.

Disorder of drug misuse is generally associated with an ADHD diagnosis in adults. A research conducted at the Long Island Jewish Medical Center and the NY State Psychiatric Institute found that, when tested as adults, hyperactive boys with ADHD displayed 12 percent antisocial personality disorder and misuse of non-alcoholic drugs, compared with 3 percent of controls.

Risk of ADHD Persistence into Adolescence

Risk factors for development of ADHD in adolescence include a inherited family propensity to ADHD, psychosocial distress and parental conflict exposure, and co-morbidity with disorders of behaviour, mood and anxiety. In the prevention of substance abuse disorders in adults with chronic ADHD, psychosocial therapy and adequate treatment at an early age are clearly important.

ADHD and Risk of Early Cigarette Smoking

ADHD is a significant risk factor for early smoking of cigarettes in children and adolescents, particularly when untreated or associated with disorder of the behavior. Latest findings at Massachusetts General Hospital, Boston, show that children treated with stimulants have a 72 percent lower chance of consuming cigarettes in adolescence and later on. The starting age or duration of stimulant therapy had no effect on the risk of smoking cigarettes.

Neurological Basis for Obsessive Compulsive Disorder

Obsessive compulsive disorder (OCD), commonly known as an anxiety neurosis, has recently been associated with anatomical defects in the basal ganglia. In a study at the Western Psychiatric Center, Pittsburgh University, PA, MRI scans of 19 children aged 7–18 years showed substantially reduced volumes of striatal basal ganglia with a recent onset of OCD. Reduced striatal volume associated with OCD symptom severity; the smaller the basal ganglia, the more extreme the symptoms. Such results contrast with the acute enlargement of the basal ganglia that associated with acute OCD exacerbation and tics in a 12-year-old boy observed by MRI at the National Institute of Mental Health, Bethesda, MD. The symptoms accompanied a streptococcal throat infection, and treatment resulted in decreased basal ganglia size and decreased OCD and tic symptoms. Basic changes in the cerebrum that connect with seriousness of side effects bolster an endogenous reason for OCD, however recommend increasingly more indisputable research.

Other Comorbid Disorders Associated with ADHD

Many of the conditions often associated with ADHD are developmental control disorder, learning disabilities, language impairment, tics, Tourette syndrome, anxiety disorders and headache. Their identification and care is key to effective ADHD management. Some researchers find sleep disruption to be a comorbid and causative factor while others underestimate a substantial link with ADHD.

Asperger's Disorder and ADHD

Asperger's syndrome is classified as a subgroup of Autistic Spectrum Disorder (ASD) or PDD. ADHD and Asperger syndrome are often comorbid, despite the ADHD diagnostic DSM-IV criteria which exclude PDD. Many children with ADHD can experience an additional comorbid PDD syndrome. Asperger's condition (high functioning ASD) DSM-IV parameters are summarized as follows:

- Deficiency of social contact.

- Limited repetitive and stereotyped behavioral patterns, preferences, and behaviors

- Serious impairments in the social, occupational, or other functional areas.

- No delay in the growth of languages.

- No delay in the development of cognitions.

- No other widespread developmental condition.

Asperger's syndrome's hallmark diagnostic criteria include a formal objective way of thinking, and an inability to identify and understand human emotions and connections. The difficulties in conversation range from stilted speech to almost robotic manner. Abnormal problems include toy cars, insects, fungi, pesticides, baby abuse, ritualistic drawings and excessive orderliness. Asperger's syndrome may overlap with or occur at the same time as Tourette's syndrome, and attention deficit disorder.

Symptoms that may be confused with ADHD are associated with learning disorders, including average or higher intelligence, especially in the areas of vocabulary, spelling, reading and visual memory. The neurological test shows symptoms of motor incoordination and non-specific EEGs. A genetic factor is suspected but no specific organic pathology is known.

The unusual personality and communication difficulties are the manifestations of Asperger's syndrome which clearly distinguish this psychiatric disorder from ADHD. In children with high verbal intelligence who do poorly at school, both academically and socially, and who display speech and language disturbances, tics, motor clumsiness, and stereotyped gestures such as excessive hand flapping, Asperger's syndrome should be considered.

In a sample of 52 affected children neurologically tested at the University of Gothenburg, Sweden, numerous biological causes for autism and autistic disorders were discovered. The EEG was 50 per cent abnormal and the CT scan revealed 25 per cent structural brain abnormalities.

The evaluation of pediatric neurology is critical in children with autistic symptoms, and EEG and CT / MRI may be indicated in selected patients. Biological abnormalities in children with signs believed to be mainly psychological and emotionally dependent may be discovered.

Sleep Disorders and ADHD

ADHD-related sleep disorders often include restless legs syndrome / periodic limb movements, rhythmic motion disturbance (rocking of the body and head banging), and parasomnia such as sleepwalking, sleep terrors, and disturbing arousals. Increased correlations between ADHD and hypersomnia such as narcolepsy and sleep apnea are also documented. Parents are to be asked about their sleep patterns.

Researchers at Chapel Hill, Carrboro, NC, University of North Carolina, examined the relationship between ADHD and parent-reported sleep issues in preschoolers aged 2–5 years. 193 children had high scores and 114 low scores out of 1,073 parents who completed the Child Development Checklist. None of the hyperactive-impulsive or inattentive symptoms of ADHD were particularly linked to issues identified by parents including sleep assistance, parasomnia or dyssomnia. Daytime sleepiness was linked to inattentive symptomatology.

A study of 412 elementary schoolchildren aged 6–12 at Penn State College of Medicine, Hershey, PA, found that overnight polysomnograph sleep scores were not related to academic performance. Conversely, IQ and neuropsychological test scores were strong achievement predictors. Children with and without issues with sleep did not vary in signs of achievement, IQ and ADHD.

CHAPTER EIGHT

Methods of Management of ADHD

The treatment of the child with ADHD includes many approaches and disciplines. This include parents, teachers, counselors, and doctors in attendance. Even in the preschool years, the parents, and particularly the mother, can be the first to draw attention to the issue. In general, the teacher raises concerns about the inattention, hyperactivity and impulsive actions of a child in kindergarten or first grade. The psychologist gets involved either on teacher recommendation or after consultation with the psychiatrist. The adult neurologist, pediatric neurologist, or child psychiatrist is usually consulted to confirm the diagnosis and monitor the medical care management.

Stimulant medicines may have the most notable and prompt beneficial effects in treating ADHD, but without family counseling, behavioral modification, and remedial education, drugs alone will only have a partial and sometimes transitory value. The practitioner is in the best position to ensure that this so-called multimodal approach to ADHD treatment is pursued, as the patient and parents are observed at regular intervals to monitor the effects of the drug and to update prescriptions. Documents will be made available to the physician at follow-up assessments by students, psychologist, and counselor.

American Academy of Pediatrics Clinical Practice Guidelines

Two sets of guidelines include suggestions for evaluating and diagnosing ADHD in children of school age (AAP, 2000) and treating ADHD (AAP, 2001). The Guidance on Diagnosis lists the following recommendations:

1. An ADHD assessment should be undertaken in a 6–12-year-old child with inattention, hyperactivity, impulsiveness, academic underperformance, or behavioral problems;

2. The child will follow the Mental Disorders Diagnostic and Statistical Manual, 4th edition of the ADHD criteria;

3. Evidence of ADHD should be collected directly from parents or caregivers about the core symptoms of ADHD in various environments, length of symptoms and degree of disability in function;

4. Evidence of ADHD should be collected directly from teacher in the classroom;

5. Related (coexisting) disorders need to be evaluated;

6. There may be other screening measures reported for similar learning disorders or mental illness.

The AAP Guidance on Care recommends:

1. ADHD is a recurrent disorder that the clinician should recognize;

2. Specify goal goals for strategic guidance;

3. Recommend medicine and/or behavioral stimulant therapy to enhance the desired outcomes;

4. Clinicians ought to assess the first finding, utilization of suitable medications and nearness of coinciding conditions when the chose administration has not met target results;

5. Periodic monitoring of the medication results per office visit every 3–6 months;

6. When one stimulant is not functioning at the maximum possible dosage, prescribe another.

Studies of adherence to the AAP Guidelines showed an overall response rate of 60%, but daily use of all diagnostic components was recorded by only 26%. Some physicians used non-recommended diagnostic modalities for regular assessments – continuous performance monitoring, neuroimaging, and laboratory testing (e.g. thyroid, lead, or iron). The majority (66.6 percent) of respondents reported daily drug use and 81 percent titrated the first month dose of medication; 53 percent reported routine follow-up visits, 3–4 times per year. A plurality (53 per cent) of physicians have suggested behavioral therapy. Half of respondents indicated that insurers had minimal coverage for assessing and treating ADHD, and 32 per cent indicated insufficient community access to mental health services.

Some groups have developed a protocol to ensure that educators and physicians cooperate. School staff are required to provide the following:

(a) Vision and hearing screening;
(b) Teacher conduct rating scales (e.g., Vanderbilt, Conner, or Achenbach);
(c) Speech / language assessment when specified;
(d) Intelligence screening and achievement testing;
(e) Complete intelligence testing when specified;
(f) Consider the need for an individualized education plan (IEP, special education) and
(g) Use contact methods to exchange reactions to the drug.

The AAP Committee on Quality Improvement and ADHD reviewed the current literature for the purpose of creating a guide to evidence-based clinical practice for the treatment of ADHD in the school-age. The evidence clearly supports the use of stimulant drugs to treat the core symptoms and, to a lesser degree, to improve the functioning of ADHD adolescents. Behavioral treatment alone only has little effect on the symptoms or behavior of ADHD children. Behavioral therapy may enhance functioning in conjunction with medication, and can decrease the amount of stimulant medication.

Roles required of the Psychologist and Psychiatrist in Child Management with ADHD. There is no substantial difference in effectiveness when comparing stimulants (methylphenidate and amphetamines).

Guidelines are not meant to be the primary source of guidance for treating ADHD children. They are designed to help primary care practitioners by offering a decision-making process. These are not intended to substitute clinical judgment or set up a procedure for all children with ADHD and do not have the only acceptable solution to this issue (AAP, 2001).

Principal Forms of Therapy of ADHD

Given the drastic early effects of stimulant treatment, a single approach to treating ADHD is never fully sufficient. In addition to the medications addressed in more depth in the next chapter, the following essential clinical regimens include:

- Psychological and psychosocial therapy

148

- Parental and family counseling

- Behavioral adjustment and/or child counseling

- Remedial instruction and learning arrangements

The optimum order of adoption of these specific treatment approaches is quite dependent. Some clinicians support initial psychosocial therapy and management of behavioral changes, while doctors also tend to incorporate treatment as an effective aid to education and academic performance early on.

Psychologist and therapist Positions in Child Care with ADHD

The counselor conducts group or individual meetings of assessment, evaluation and/or therapy, and advises on class selection, behavior management, and adequate academic accommodation. The doctor diagnoses and treats with psychotherapy and medicine. Some university-based psychiatrists are psycho-pharmacologists, who are trained in drug testing and trials for ADHD and comorbid disorders.

Psychologists specialize in offering research and/or treatment, as educational or clinical psychologists. Some are qualified to provide all kinds of services. A parent can consult with a psychologist about ADHD symptoms or a learning issue as a first resort, or the physician or teacher's advice. Any child who has learning or behavioral difficulties may require a psychologist's services at some point. This can be made available via the school or mental health program, or in private.

Barkley (1997) and Millichap (1984) address the psychological impact of a disabled child on family life, peer relationships, and strategies for counselling and educating children's families with ADHD.

Doctor's Role In Helping Parents Understand And Tackle ADHD Issue

As the scientific evidence supports a neurobiological or genetic basis for ADHD, the main responsibility for the issue has moved from the parents to the brain of the child and a neurochemical or structural brain disorder. Neurological evidence has dismissed the argument by sociologists and others that ADHD reflects a "deviating activity," primarily under the influence of the child-parent-child relationship. The findings of scientific research have supported the "medicalisation" of ADHD and its diagnosis as a "illness."

The doctor describes the factors considered to underlie the ADHD symptoms and orders tests to rule out possible causes as necessary. Although the practitioner is responsible for treatment and care supervision, parents need to consider the effect of child-family involvement and remedial education on therapy interventions successfully. The parents are equally responsible for educating themselves in their role in managing the child in the home. Parental discord and hardship to the family community can worsen the ADHD symptoms and reduce the efficacy of medical care.

Useful Parental Advice in ADHD Treatment

Living with a hyperactive child requires patience and empathy between parents, siblings and neighbours. The following ideas can be considered helpful for parents:

- Avoid repetition of "no" and "don't."

- Use affirmation whenever necessary and promote positive behaviors to create self-confidence and self-esteem;

- Find an interest in education or sport which motivates and encourages and supports a child.

- Talk slowly and quietly;

- Present assignments or errands, one at a time.

- Strengthen verbal requests or explanations by using written or picture signs.

- Promote a regular, quiet homework schedule, mealtime, playtime and bedtime.

- Avoid formal restaurant meals if noisy and arguable.

- Make playmates less boisterous and discourage disruptive activities.

- Seek the assistance of a family counselor or psychologist, especially if the ADHD is compounded by an opposition defiant or a disorder of behavior.

Motivational Strategies Stressed In Therapy and Preparation Programs For The Parents

Perhaps most significant of all those parental strategies is the focus on encouragement.

Parents frequently wonder why their child should concentrate on an activity like Nintendo or a favorite television show while displaying in-school diversion and inattentiveness. The response relates to the essence of attention and the effect of demands and disturbances on the environment.

The learning process will fall into four categories:

1. Goals-consciousness,

2. Look out,

3. Selectiveness, and

4. Too much tenacity.

The child with ADHD appears to be hyper-vigilant but has deficiencies in selection and treatment. There is an impediment to the discrimination of essential from unessential stimuli.

Attention can be guided by situational demands and goal-consciousness or motivation.

Through seeking fun opportunities and offering encouragement and affirmation, parents may inspire the child to follow the correct interests. Excellent motivating resources are biographies of famous people who have overcome adversity to excel in their chosen field of endeavour.

Winston Spencer Churchill, who by his outstanding leadership and oratory rescued Britain from the tyranny of Hitler's Germany, and later wrote a best-selling British Empire History, had signs of ADHD, speech impediment, and learning disability as a child (Churchill, 1930). In his autobiography, My Early Life, Churchill wrote: "Overall, my school days have greatly discouraged me." "It is not pleasant to feel so outstripped and left behind at the very beginning of the race." He was surprised to hear his teacher predict when he left school, "With a confidence that I could see no foundation that I should be able to make my way right."

A simple word of praise or a teacher's note of trust leaves its impression on a child with academic difficulties for life. But Churchill did make his way perfect. He was Great Britain's Prime Minister, and a world leader. Several famous people, including Churchill, have been recorded suffering from learning disabilities during childhood. Among those identified as dyslexic are Thomas Edison, Albert Einstein, President Woodrow Wilson and Governor Nelson Rockefeller, and their names are indelibly written in historical documents.

Nancy Millichap refers in the book on dyslexia (Millichap and Millichap, 1986), to papers about Thomas Edison's childhood and other historical figures. His teacher diagnosed Thomas Edison, the inventor, as mentally ill, his father thought he was crazy, he never learned to spell and his spelling was appalling until the time of his manhood. Physicist and Nobel Prize laureate Albert Einstein did not speak until he was four, nor read until nine. Her teachers and his father found Einstein to be backward. U.S. President Woodrow Wilson did not learn his letters until he was nine, or he learned to read until he was eleven., The former governor of New York State, Nelson A. Rockefeller and vice-president of the United States, recalled his struggles as a dyslexic child in an essay in the 1976 TV Guide, entitled "Don't Embrace Anyone's Opinion That You Are Lazy, Dumb, or Retarded." Classes and teachers for children with reading impairments were not available in his day. Nowadays, with our new understanding of dyslexia and other learning disorders, a child's academic difficulties will have a lighter burden and better opportunities.

The Child's Involvement in Management of ADHD

Every doctor, parent and teacher has a role to play in treating the child with ADHD. In patients with mental, mood or anxiety disorders, resistant to simpler interventions, advanced clinical or psychiatric therapy is required. Behavior management therapy using incentives as an alternative to medical care can be beneficial.

The physician should describe the essence of the drug condition and its function. Methylphenidate (Ritalin R) is used as an educational aid, to help focus and reduce distractibility, not specifically to change behaviour. While the interruption therapy procedure is debatable, medications may be removed at weekends and on holidays. Exceptions to drug holidays involve children involved in school or homework tasks, and impulse activity that presents a health and well-being threat.

Parents should celebrate performance, accept disappointment and avoid unnecessary or harsh criticism, but with adequate and consistent discipline, patience should be balanced with. Teachers explain the complexity of the learning challenge with the aid of the psychologist, stressing the strengths and explaining how shortcomings can be rectified through preparation. The secret to success is positive mindset on the part of parents, teachers and all professionals.

Behavior Modification Therapy: Methods and Results

Modification of behavior is a systemic type of environmental structuring, based on the premise that behavior is regulated either by pleasurable or denied gratification. A child is believed to change actions in order to receive incentives and to escape limits, denials or reprimands.

A program of incentives, denials, or reprimands is developed and fully explained to the child and to all family members. There should be presence of both parents at home and teachers in classroom. Effective or beneficial behavior is rewarded and reinforced positively, and a negative reinforcement of bad or unwanted actions. Positive reinforcement is generally favored and stressed although it can require immediate reprimands as a more aggressive behavioral intervention. The tokens used as positive reinforcement are provided to the child and are exchanged for goods or services according to a tariff and value schedule. Time outs in a quiet room and TV viewing time rejection or limitation are examples of constructive feedback and the effects of inacceptable behaviour.

Classroom reinforcer requires individual focus, immediate and consistent recognition for successful performance, and responsibility for specific assignments and incentives. Repressions should be performed immediately, and not delayed if possible. A research by the Emory University on the reactions of ADHD children to behavioral intervention alone and in conjunction with stimulant medication has shown that immediate teacher reprimands can achieve results comparable to those of stimulants. These behavioral interventions, however, are labor intensive and not available to the majority of children with ADHD. Additionally, treatment will obviate the need for intensive therapeutic therapy for certain children.

Modification of actions on the part of parents, teachers and therapists takes time, persistence and some compulsiveness. When the scheme is to be implemented reliably and uniformly over an prolonged period of time, the thorough explanations needed in practice are generally beyond the reach of most physicists. Parents interested in the method should receive professional assistance through the local community mental health center or a psychiatrist or private consultant.

In practice alone behavioral therapy is rarely successful, but it can be of benefit in conjunction with medication. Individual counselling with a psychologist or social worker is usually required in children with ADHD complicated by ODD or CD.

Teacher and school system position in ADHD management

The instructor is also the first person to consider inattention, hyperactivity and impulsiveness of a child and suspect an ADHD diagnosis. The instructor may complete ADHD and behavioral questionnaires after discussion with the parents, such as the Conner, McCarney, Quay and Peterson, or the Vanderbilt rating scales. Depending on the incapacity of a child to work satisfactorily in the usual classroom and the outcomes of the questionnaires, more assessment can be carried out by a school psychologist or instructor of learning impairment. A consultation may be recommended with the child's pediatrician or a pediatric neurologist.

Reasonable changes will be made in class selection and school instruction after parent – teacher conferences are completed. Learning disabilities found by psychiatric testing should be remedied using special educational approaches. Kids with ADD have educational rights protected by federal law.

Federal Legislation on the Treatment of Children with ADHD

Two federal laws provide adequate education for children with ADHD who are enrolled in federally funded public schools or private schools. Which are the 1973 Rehabilitation Act, Persons with

Disabilities Act (IDEA), and Section 504. In a "Policy Clarification Document" dated September 16, 1991, the Department of Education states that under Part B of the Concept, students with ADD are eligible for special education and related services only on the basis of their ADD when it substantially impairs educational or learning results.

As with other disorders included under the Proposal, it must be determined that the ADD has substantial adverse effects on the educational performance of a child. The assessment of multidisciplinary teams may be appropriate to assess whether special education and/or related services are needed. For children seeking resource room support or instruction, an Individual Education Plan (IEP) is planned.

While the IDEA requires a child with ADD to be eligible for special services with a learning problem, Section 504 covers children with behavioral problems such as hyperactivity, not complicated by learning disabilities.

The American with Disabilities Act (ADA), 1990, provides additional legislative provisions for children attending public schools and private non-religious schools with ADDs. A local chapter of CHADD (Children and Adults with Attention Deficit Disorders) will provide information to parents if special education services are needed.

Classroom Hospitality for ADHD and Learning Disorders

The Federal Government Department of Education suggests classroom accommodations and remedial education that include the following examples:

- Structured learning environment

- Individualized homework assignments

- Written as well as verbal instructions

- Extended time for tests

- Access to tape recorders and computers

- Behavior modification techniques

The parent should meet with the teacher in order to discuss and implement the recommended changes in a child's curriculum. This "individual educational plan or program (IEP)" typically includes the parent.

Public School Places of Special Education for Children with ADHD

The different special education services are graded according to the nature and form of learning and/or behavioral disability of the child, from moderate to severe, as follows:

1. Classroom daily and part-time tutoring,

2. Standard classroom plus part-time resource space, daily for 1/2–2 h.

3. For other subjects, part-time learning disability class plus resource room and mainstreaming or integration into daily class.

4. Class with full-time learning disability (LD), or behavioral disorder (ED).

5. Full-time class "educable mentally disabled" (for children with 60–80 IQ and not graded as ADHD or LD).

The benefits of resource room and intellectual disability class are the small scale that allows for more individual focus, and teacher staffing with special intellectual disorder credentials. The downside of these groups is the stigma of early-age labeling and isolation of the child from peers. However, if the aim is communicated individually to the child and to the class and parents, then the special education will soon be recognized if academic achievements result.

Professional Support Services in Public Schools

Specialized support services made available for children attending public schools with ADHD include:

- **School psychologist**: When a child is considered to have a learning disability, the counselor is called upon to administer individual comprehension, vision, and reading assessments, and to determine social-emotional factors that underlie behavioral problems. The independently conducted psychological assessment differs from the performance assessments (Iowa, Stanford, or California) that are provided to a group at more frequent intervals by the school or learning disorder instructor. Families often get confused about the counselor and the LD teacher conducting tasks and tests.

- **Social Worker**: The school social worker can provide behavioral problems child counseling services, and emotional support and reassurance for those dealing with issues like divorce or peer pressure.

- **Faculty nurse**: The school nurse also assumes responsibility for administering medicine at lunchtime, recording any side effects, and maintains reports of necessary immunizations, and tests of vision and hearing.

- **Instructor in remedial reading**: For individual or group guidance and preparation, children with dyslexia or lesser degrees of reading difficulty may be referred to the read specialist.

- **Speaking pathologist**: Speech and language tests are carried out by the school staff if the comprehension and/or expressive language skills of a child are impaired. The speech-pathologist often offers patient or group therapy.

- **Career psychologist**: Guidance counselors are especially available in high schools. They help students choose schools, jobs, and universities. For lower grades a guidance counselor may assist with tutors and recommendations on placement in grades or special schools.

- **Exercising trainer**: Occupational therapy (OT) interventions for children with ADHD exacerbated by motor incoordination are also recommended. OT can also help promote gross coordination and encourage children to take part in group physical activities.

Guidelines for a private or rehabilitation school for children with ADHD

Private educational facilities for ADHD children are either day schools, or internships. Private day school or rehabilitation school may be necessary when the system of public schools can not offer sufficient special educational services. The boarding school may be the perfect placement for the boy, who needs special care 24 hours a day in a well-structured environment.

Children with learning and language disabilities may not show the anticipated rate of improvement in standard public school placements, and may require more comprehensive and individualized teaching programs. The small teacher-pupil ratio in private schools is an advantage, but it is also prohibitive to charge the fees needed to have this optimum placement.

Tutoring rRle in Children's Education with ADHD

The most versatile and least visible way of offering special education is individual tutoring. The professional tutor will also assume the role of counselor and advisor in addition to supplementing school teaching, improving self-confidence and allaying a child's anxieties about school success. If a mentor is recommended the decision should be made if necessary in consultation with the main teacher in the classroom. That allows for consistency between classroom work and homework.

CHAPTER NINE

Medications for ADHD

Medicines, especially stimulants to the central nervous system, are an essential part of ADHD care. The use of stimulants in children for treating hyperactive behavior was first identified in 1937, starting with amphetamines. Regulated methylphenidate (Ritalin R) trials in the 1960s demonstrated sign-nificant benefits without any significant side effects. In addition to a decrease in physical activity, there was greater emphasis and attention and better schoolwork, grades and social behaviour (Conners and Eisenberg, 1963). Methylphenidate supports learning in low to moderate doses, without impairing imaginative or flexible thought. The effectiveness of stimulant medicine in treating ADHD has stood the test of time.

Continuing work has given answers to many of the questions of parents, and has verified the efficacy and safety of long-term drug use.

Stimulant Medications Recommended for Treatment of ADHD

Ritalin R is the ideal central nervous stimulant for the treatment of ADHD, or its generic version, methylphenidate. Ritalin-SR and ConcertaTM are prolonged-release, long-acting methylphenidate preparations. Bradley (1937), who first employed Benzedrine (D, L-amphetamine) and later, in 1950, Dexedrine (D-amphetamine), is generally credited with the earliest recorded usage of stimulant drugs for hyperactive children. Benzedrine is no longer available, and Dexedrine is largely substituted by Adderall R, a mixture of amphetamines which seems to have superior properties to D-amphetamine alone. Lisdexamfetamine, a new amphetamine sold under the brand name Vyvanse R, has a slower onset of action than Dexedrine, with peak effect at 2.5 h and activity period up to 12 hours. Cylert R (pemoline) is another long-acting stimulant, but it is no longer available due to reported liver toxicity.

In action, variations in brand potency, trade preparation, Ritalin R, and the generic version, methylphenidate, are commonly encountered. Replacing the Ritalin brand for the generic preparation may result in a change in efficacy. A lack of reaction to the generic methylphenidate would cause a brand review.

Paradoxical Calming Effect of Stimulant Medications

A psychostimulant medicine has the primary function of increasing focus and alertness. The amphetamines structurally resemble neurotransmitters, catecholamines which facilitate the passage of impulses from one nerve cell to another. They are thought to increase catecholamine production in neuronal synapses, resulting in neurotransmitter accumulation, norepinephrine and dopamine, and serotonin at higher doses. The D-isomer is a more active stimulant than the L-isomer and has a stronger effect on dopaminergic transmission. Methylphenidate is structurally similar to amphetamine, and a reuptake inhibitor for dopamine and catecholamine. It raises neurotransmitter production at the synaptic cleft, but enhancing serotonin transmission through methylphenidate is less than with amphetamines.

The brain has motor pathways both rewarding and inhibitory, regulated by the neurochemical transmitters. A neurotransmitter deficiency may weaken the inhibition and allow for excessive motor activity. In principle, brain dopamine and norepinephrine are absent in children with ADHD. The so-called paradoxical psychostimulant calming effect may be associated with an increase and correction in the levels of these neurotransmitter chemicals in the brain, restoring the role of inhibitory pathways. Though maintaining and increasing the degree of alertness, these chemical effects are thought to normalize motor activity.

The metabolic mechanisms in catecholamine production and amphetamine activity are as follows:

TYROSINE > DOPA > DOPAMINE > NOREPINEPHRINE

Chemicals and cofactors, including pyridoxal phosphate and ascorbate, are associated with those components. Inside the nerve terminals, catecholamines are put away vesicles. Amphetamines dislodge catecholamines from the capacity vesicles, permitting synapses to spill from the nerve terminals.

Another option or supplement to the neurochemical hypothesis depends on the neuroanatomic situation of the psychostimulant activity and its impact on the frontal flap, a locale with an inhibitory engine movement sway.

Specific Benefits of Stimulant Medication in ADHD

The kid is less distractible, has a more extended capacity to focus, and is less forceful and hasty, notwithstanding a progressively situated conduct. Better visual vision, eye-hand coordination, drawing and penmanship, facilitate homework more, and advance the accomplishment of better evaluations.

In one of the most punctual controlled viability preliminaries of Ritalin R, performed at Children's Memorial Hospital, NWU, Chicago, 68 percent of 30 youngsters with ADHD earned advantages over a preliminary span of 3 weeks. Neuropsychological testing showed appreciation, visual memory and eye-hand coordination changes. An ensuing investigation of the writing, and investigations of an aggregate of 337 kids in seven separate Ritalin preliminaries, found a 83 percent expansion by and large.

Subsequent studies of methylphenidate (MPH) trials and other central nervous stimulants involving nearly 5,000 children continued to show positive response in 70–80 per cent of topics. Improve hyperactive behavior, self-esteem, learning, and functioning socially and in the family. Results of MPH on comorbid disorders of opposition and behavior are mixed, with some investigators documenting a lack of response, while others pointing to an increase in the ratings of teacher behavior. MPH typically has a greater level of positive effects on ADHD than on oppositional comorbid disorders and behavior disorders. Children who do not respond to medication need to put greater focus on behavioral therapy and counseling for parents.

Patients with ADHD Most Likely to Respond to Stimulant Drugs

Methylphenidate (MPH) treatment is the well on the way to help youngsters who are generally forceful, indiscreet, and distractible. In Millichap (1973), these indicators of the reaction to MPH were accounted for and checked in consequent investigations in Barkley et al. (1991) and Handen et al. (1994). While MPH can be proposed without hyperactivity and impulsivity in a kid with ADD, an answer is progressively plausible when the youngster is hyperactive, as well.

Helpful indicators of a positive long haul reaction are the clinical evaluation of the degree of ADHD and progress revealed after a solitary portion of MPH. In 46 youngsters with ADHD treated at the University of Utrecht, The Netherlands, prescient elements for reaction to MPH were inspected. MPH standardized school conduct in one portion of understudies, and home conduct in 33%. Indicators of response to MPH incorporated a high remainder of knowledge, outrageous heedlessness and absence of tension. Positive social changes, estimated after a solitary 10 mg portion of MPH by the Abbreviated Conners 'rating scales, were prescient of proceeded with progress following a month of treatment.

Inventiveness and Flexibility of Thinking During Treatment with Methylphenidate

Some parents are worried that a medication given to improve concentrate power and control impulsivity can at the same time reduce a child's thought ability and flexibility. Researchers studying creativity effects, assessed by the Torrance nonverbal thought test, found that methylphenidate (MPH) in 19 boys with ADHD had no negative effects on creative thinking. Impulsive power is independent of the imagination. In addition, experiments using acute, single MPH doses of 0.3 and 0.6 mg enhanced versatility of thought and speed and accuracy of processing information. MPH does not affect the imagination and versatility of learning of an infant in low to moderate doses.

Connection of the Dose of Methylphenidate to the Response of ADHD Symptoms

The methylphenidate reaction (MPH) is portion related, especially for assignments that require consideration. Lower dosages (0.3 mg/kg) improve intellectual execution and learning capacity while higher portions (1.0 mg/kg) that debilitate adapting however improve social conduct, as indicated by one examination (Sprague and Sleator, 1977). A later report indicated that MPH's helpful consequences for scholastic execution didn't contrast with measurements yet with the bigger portion, social changes were supported further. In the first part of the day, the lower portion (0.3 mg/kg) made both scholarly and social changes that were never again present toward the evening. A higher morning portion (1.0 mg/kg) was trailed by tenacious social changes, and by the evening scholarly increases evaporated. Symptoms remembering an expansion for beat rate and circulatory strain have just been seen with the more noteworthy measurements.

Ongoing investigations have considered the impacts of MPH at four unique degrees of portion: 5, 10, 15 and 20 mg. The consequences for the working of the study hall were identified with the portion of MPH, remembering for task center, work fulfillment and educator appraisals. Employment exactness was improved at all portion levels, and undertaking culmination at single dosages over 5 mg was altogether more noteworthy. In kids who didn't react to low-portion MPH, the focal point of consideration was delicate to increases in the portion, while conduct and scholastic accomplishment were not improved with bigger dosages.

These all around controlled research examines demonstrate that littler dosages of MPH can bolster both scholarly execution and activity, and are commonly desirable over a solitary bigger portion, however the impact is fleeting and the portion must be rehashed to look after adequacy. In attempting to decide an ideal portion for every individual youngster, the time of activity on scholarly, psychological, and conduct execution must be estimated.

The impacts on the fixation and learning of two distinct dosages (0.3 and 0.8 mg/kg) of methylphenidate (MPH) in 23 kids matured 7–11 with ADHD were surveyed at the Scottish Rite Children's Medical Center, Atlanta, GA. Constant adequacy execution was improved with low-portion MPH and lack of caution estimated by the quantity of commission blunders was diminished. In nonverbal learning and memory undertakings, the simple degree of assignment execution was improved similarly with either portion of MPH, though the hard errand was done well just with the high portion.

Low doses of MPH gain attention and impulsivity but higher doses may be needed to enhance retention and retrieval of complex nonverbal information. Cognitive function and actions are susceptible to stimulant medication, but doses for each patient must be individualized and titrated.

MPH is normally administered two or three times a day, after breakfast, at school lunchtime, and at 3–4 in the afternoon if appropriate. Usually, the initial dose is 5 mg, two or three times daily, irrespective of the child's age or weight, at 5 years of age and above. No dose – response varies with body weight.

If a dose increase is deemed appropriate then amounts should be low, 2.5 mg daily, at intervals not less than 1 week. Doses greater than 10 mg, two or three times daily, are usually not effective in my experience, and are frequently followed by unnecessary side effects. In extreme cases, a child can need 15 or 20 mg in the morning for optimum learning results. In general, if small or moderate doses of MPH are ineffective, the diagnosis and treatment choice should be reassessed, and some alternative form of stimulant or drug change should be considered.

MPH Dosage Plan Twice Daily or Three Times a Day

Methylphenidenidate has suggested activity and learning outcomes in the classroom twice daily for children with ADHD but not at home. A three-time daily dosing schedule will allow homework assignments to be completed and will foster relationships between parent and child. The twice daily dose schedule may be ideal for lower grades of schooling, but in higher grades with a heavier academic load, an additional dose of MPH may be needed at 3 or 4, given there is no sleeping habit disturbance. Additionally, the third dose can prevent any effects of MPH rebound experienced upon school return.

A 5-week, placebo-controlled combination study at the University of Chicago compared the effectiveness and side effects of twice daily (bid) and triple daily (tid) MPH dosing schedules in 25 ADHD boys (mean dose: 8 mg [0.3 mg / kg]). Three times regular dose provided greater gain on Conners 'parent and teacher rating scales than the bid system, and the occurrence of side effects, like insomnia, did not alter.

A placebo-controlled study at the Hospital for Sick Children in Toronto, Canada, of 91 children receiving MPH, titrated to 0.7 mg / kg twice daily over a 4-month span, found symptoms of ADHD and comorbid oppositional disorder improved in school but not when they returned home. Rebound side effects observed by parents included depression, personality change, irritability, withdrawal lethargy, aggressive activity and mild mania.

Children in the Toronto study, receiving comparatively high doses of MPH twice daily, reported regular rebound symptoms on returning home in the afternoon, while in the Chicago study, a three-fold daily schedule and lower doses of MPH were correlated with consistent change in behavior rating scales and far less side effect. In addition, a parent-child conflict-free evening and a satisfactorily completed homework task, resulting from a third dose of MPH, will contribute to increased self-esteem and stronger success in the classroom.

Methylphenidate Protection and Efficacy In Pre-School Children With ADHD

Most of methylphenidate trials in ADHD is performed in children 5 years of age and older. Families of pre-school children with ADHD are often encouraged to focus on behavior modification therapy, a treatment technique that is rarely successful in itself. Owing to FDA limitations and lack of clinically monitored trials in children under 6 years of age, doctors are hesitant to recommend stimulants for younger children. In the following research it is shown that MPH in conservative doses will support learning and behavior in preschool children.

The Perspective of Child Stimulant Medication and Its Effect on Peer Relationships

At the University of Ottawa, Canada, 31 children aged 4–6 years with ADHD and comorbid oppositional disorder were treated with MPH (0.3 and 0.5 mg / kg twice daily) in a double-blind, placebo-controlled trial.Significant results were made during therapy with MPH on a cognitive test (number of correct answers to the Gordon Vigilance Task), parent ratings of child behaviour, and tests assessing the ability to complete a paper-and-pencil assignment. Improved performance during therapy with MPH was also reported on impulsivity-hyperactivity tests and behaviour. With the higher dose of MPH, side effects, stomachache, headache, anxiety and depression increased in frequency and severity.

MPH Effectiveness in ADHD Adolescents

The signs of ADHD in teenagers are almost comparable with those in childhood, and the effectiveness and side effects of methylphenidate (MPH) are similar in both age groups as well. The dosage of MPH should not be raised automatically, based on age and weight gains. Patients with ADHD who experience symptoms increasing in high school will undergo psychosocial therapy and/or tutoring until recommending that the stimulant dose increase.

In a longitudinal follow-up study of 16 patients enrolled in summer treatment services, the efficacy of MPH, 0.3 mg / kg, in ADHD was measured during childhood and adolescence at the Western Psychiatric Institute, University of Pittsburgh, PA. Of 12 objective metrics of academic achievement and social conduct, as well as counselor and instructor scores, only 3 showed substantial improvements in MPH sensitivity from childhood to teenage.

In childhood and adolescence stimulant therapy is similarly beneficial for ADHD, given the atmosphere and behaviors remain constant. If drug misuse in adolescence is a issue it is independent of

ADHD. In certain centers bupropion therapy, which has a lower risk for misuse, is replaced with stimulant medicine (Riggs, 1998). When drug misuse is suspected, the other alternative treatment is the tamper proof, longer-acting OROS formulation of methylphenidate (Concerta R) or the non-stimulant, atomoxetine (Strattera R).

Conclusion

A number of common Attention Deficit Hyperactivity Disorder books suggest that this is not a concern but a blessing that brings different abilities to people with ADHD. But if ADHD is a blessing then why do people with ADHD have so many negative social statistics?

On average, people with ADHD are more likely to become involved in major car crashes, are more likely to have unplanned pregnancies, are more likely to misuse drugs, and are less likely to keep a work down. When ADHD is such a blessing then it is a blessing without which other people will be better off.

The ADHD is a gift concept focused on a distorted view of people living with ADHD. As ADHD researcher Russell Barkley points out, most common adult ADHD books and articles concentrate on ADHD among well-educated, middle-class people with moderate ADHD rates-just the kind of people who are likely to read ADHD books and seek support. There's no question that a high percentage of these people are smart or creative-but that doesn't mean they have those attributes because they have ADHD. It could only be that they happen to be smart or talented people come from families that are fairly stable and successful.

There are also individuals from poor, low-income families on the other side of the equation, who have ADHD and are never officially diagnosed. And some researchers claim that more than half of the U.S. prison population has ADHD. That means there's a huge segment of the ADHD population that is still struggling to get through, but this category is rarely mentioned in common ADHD books. The extremely impaired side of the condition is often only discussed on the subject in the scientific literature.

Also, there is a smaller community of people with ADHD who are silent underdogs. Typically, these individuals have the inattentive form of ADHD, and are more likely to be underemployed. These are often more likely to experience depression or anxiety disorders, and are more likely to live as adults with their parents. To this party, ADHD is not much a blessing either. Unassuming under-supporters of inattentional ADHD, however, are not much discussed in ADHD books because they do not appear to draw attention to themselves and are less likely to seek assistance.

Many who say ADHD is a blessing often suggest that highly creative people with ADHD are. The reality here is harder to learn. Those who are particularly imaginative in popular culture appear to have a reputation for being fragmented and absent-minded. Because creative thinking, such as signs of ADHD, appear to be associated in some areas of the brain with slower brain-wave states, some correlation between creativity and ADHD is likely. Though, it is important to note that there are a lot of creative people that don't have ADHD, so ADHD isn't an absolute creativity necessity.

ADHD is a condition which certain individuals have and which, depending on the individual's ability and conditions, may or may not be a serious issue. It is also important to note that you do not have ADHD, it is something you have. Be proud of the good qualities and abilities, but don't equate them with the issues associated with ADHD. Doing so would just make it easier to control the condition, and objectively evaluate the strengths and weaknesses.

CPSIA information can be obtained
at www.ICGtesting.com
Printed in the USA
LVHW050345120121
676187LV00005B/291